FULL BELLY METER

Weight Loss System

Katherine Giesbrecht

First paperback edition, 2016
First printing, 2016
Publisher: Katherine Giesbrecht
Library & Archives Canada
ISBN: 978-0-9949185-0-5
http://www.fullbellymeter.com ©

Photo Attributions: Depositphotos www.depositphotos.com
Contributors: saje/depositphotos.com: 7380photostudio/depositphotos.com

DEDICATION

This book is dedicated to my much better half Todd, such a real joy he is; who is not afraid to share together, cry together or love together forever and after, whose unlimited devotion and support and patience that rivals an elephants' memory has made me a better person today.

To my late mother Julia who would have been so proud. She would have carried my book in her purse to show everyone she knew or ran into for sure.

And lastly to my Berkley for his loving bravery and constant companionship who always has my back.

CONTENTS

CHAPTER 1

CHAPTER 2

CHAPTER 3

CHAPTER 4

CHAPTER 1

ॐ

WHY THIS SYSTEM

The Full Belly Meter System © was developed out of my own pure personal weight frustration journey. This book includes the journey, system and workbook all in one. I am a real person just like all of you and was at my wits end as you must be today. I care about your weighted feelings because I have been there and know how you feel. I am sincerely interested in you getting to your goals and what happens on your journey there. I want to share how my system is unique in how it changed my negative cognitive behaviour by replacing some negatives with positive cognitive braintraining, I call that my BadAss Belly

Braintrain behaviour technique (my system). This helped me realize with clarity how my own body weight worked and what to do about it. It is a very valuable system and just so extremely easy and it will not drain the pocketbook. This behaviour changing system helps to create a more immediate self-control from the start as well as it holds you completely accountable right from day 1 to yourself. My suggested system just totally empowers you to revamp your own browbeating weighted feelings and to make something positive for yourself that shines through into your progress like you never thought was possible. For people having had gastric bypass surgery, any weight loss surgery or medical conditions weight related, if you are pregnant, or under the legal age where you live do not use this system and you must follow your Dr's specific dietary food instructions instead. My suggested system book is about a 1 hour reading process; then you should be ready to begin. You will not need to run out to the grocery store right away. You will have a few days to gather your grocery list and whatever else you need later in the week.

Are you a weightloss seeker about ready to give up? Not! Full Belly Meter is the 'missing bridge' to get you back on track. Full Belly Meter Weight Loss System is not a diet, it is a cognitive braintrain technique or 'SYSTEM'. The ultimate self help guide to help create the 'body to brain weight loss A-Ha connection' that forces insight into where you may be going wrong even though others seem to be doing great, but not you.

Full Belly Meter is NOT the drop the pounds real quick diet. The FBM system is intended to #1. Time bridge you from a self-recognition start point that you can do from home using the system book and using a fully encompassing healthier lifestyle approach. There is also more in depth healthier bang for your nutrition-buck suggestions at our Full Belly Meter website, courses and our free or paid groups as well that is most supplemental to this book. Learn and educate yourself with us about things we feel important to lead to healthier weight loss geared to help toward the longer haul. #2 We feel this is spot on. You learn it, lose what you will from it; and then maintain it for the longer healthier haul.

It is super you are here reading this because if you had been doing everything right all these years you would not need to be here.   It is obvious something you have been doing repeatedly IS NOT WORKING for you. Before Full Belly Meter Weight Loss System; I was not achieving the weight loss A-ha moment, there was no default body system of automatic brain to body progress that I felt should have naturally just been there. I realized that a span of over twenty years passed and still I had no weight comfort zone and no weight A-ha moment. This book describes in good precise detail the system, process and steps to authors' braintrain weight loss A-ha moment that sticks like cemented glue when it was put into practice. Before I started my system I knew that I had to obtain good health to achieve good weight loss. I also knew I had to change my bad food behaviors and I had to get the biggest bang for my nutritional buck. In the beginning; I tried various things each day moving forward till my notebook became filled with hundreds of notes, but at the 30-day mark in doing this it hit me unexpectedly and the A-ha weight loss moment arrived and my system was born. Good health is more than just food in and food out, it is our whole healthy picture. It is also our bad habits we keep repeating, our genetics, our environmental factors, our belief systems, our lack of sleep, our stresses, our addictions, our medical conditions, exercise and our lack of education about healthy satiating food choices and how to eat healthier. As well, macronutrients especially sufficient protein, healthy fats, healthy carbs and saying goodbye to sugar – all key. I could have just stayed miserable and obese; blaming my Hashimoto's thyroid condition which we have all read about how thyroid and weight interact together and the news is never great.

I could also have whined about my x-ray results at the L5-S1 narrowed back disk with arthritis present and throbbing around in there making exercise on most days pretty much excruciating or impossible. I could have blamed the severe stress factors in my life for the weight gain or all of the failed attempts or tries that sort of worked but then just petered out. I could have just kept complaining about not being able to lose the extra pounds I put on from quitting smoking which omg was another approximately 10 pounds and add onto that the extra baby weight of another 20 pounds shortly thereafter. You can see the slow but sure mounting stress of extra pounds gathering after each of these significant events. I could have just given up altogether – but I did not and I am so happy now that I just pushed blindly forward realizing I needed to get healthier; and that if I gain the health I lose the weight!

My weight had eventually tipped into the 200's and that was my personal prison when I was there.   Anyone who has been there knows that feeling I am talking about and this was very impacting to me on many levels.

How many years have you been silently thinking to yourself like I did that you are just so utterly sick and tired of the fat? Just so fed up with the hills, bumps and valleys that seem surreal on your body but when you look in that mirror, there they all are staring back at you. In fact, reminding you of your unhappiness in the looking glass. I used to think about how many years I had not been able to just glance down and easily see my feet below when standing upright and how my feet kept disappearing more and more below me. I remember tallying up the years I have been unhappy with my weight and realized I just don't have that same amount of time left on this earth to fix this as I spent worrying about it. Some of you can relate to underwear, how about not being able to wear underwear properly because it rolls down the hills and valleys or just gets buried in there somewhere. I remember attending well over twenty years ago to my first weight loss class and weekly weight loss classes ongoing thereafter. I recall swallowing or drinking the newest weight loss discovery to find that if I quit my newest discovery or quit my classes instructions then my fat just magically built up and returned on its' own. I just felt like I had tried it all and could see what a rollercoaster of emotional abuse this weight loss worrying was taking as a whole toll on my mind spirit and body. It felt like being on an endless journey at sea and the captain says 'we are going south and we shall find land'; and then we head south but we never reach the land and sand that I can plant and dig my feet and toes into. However, that land is truly there somewhere yonder and I knew that there just had to be more and I was going to find it and dig my heels in and so I did.

Prior to my Full Belly Meter © system, with other plans and attempts I was able to achieve 'temporary happiness' because none of it would work on a more permanent basis for me (the caloric intake changed but not my braintrain). At that time I had not read that 90% of diets fail after the 1 to 2 year mark of going off and weight is often regained. An example of that is back in the time when a family member passed on and I took a break away from my plans and classes. I found I had to get back on the wagon, or go back and start whatever I was doing again just to get back to where I left off. This repeating behaviour happened to me I realized for over a 20 year plus span of always trying to lose weight and yo-yoing because when I was off or away the pounds came on again. And the roller coaster would yet begin again. I was somewhat happy with some successes but knew I could be happier yet if I could just make that default brain to body cognitive behaviour connection. In my younger years I did my part towards countless expensive things that I would faithfully attend, various diets, pills and fads, support groups, chat groups, gadgets, scales, buying countless cookbooks and counting stuff for years on end and you name it. There had just been no default A-ha weight loss moment connection to food verses the belly verses the poundage for me after all the pill, powder, brand pushing things.

I will give credit where credit is due because from attending all my various things and trying all that was out there that I thought would help me, I gained from this a lot of wonderful recipes and hints and tips. I met a ton of really nice good people that understood my battle and I also gained many wonderful cookbooks and insights that all just strengthen and increase the so needed weight loss education as a whole. To do my Full Belly System, I did not need to throw away all my prior acquired information, books, cookbooks etc. which is super because I not only hate to waste food but I also hate to waste my time and money.

Thinking back on the yo-yoing, I realized my problem was I always tried to follow multiple things that had just the calories all spelled out basically (no braintrain) so in fact I thought it just had to work. I realize now that I was not following my natural logical mind-body-food-cell interaction and recognition of same and not benefitting myself as much as I could. I instinctively knew inside my real deal could only happen with the A-ha moment and that A-ha moment would not trail blaze its way down from the skies and bonk me on the head because after twenty more plus years of my trying it just never happened that way. No real clarity ever presented me smack in my face like this system does to me.

I experienced from thinking out of the box and just dragging my little note book everywhere with me that 'the moment' was a whole lifestyle process that had to be learned by my brain and body. I learned from my Full Belly Meter © personal system that my weight struggle for a very large part in my personal journey had to begin and both end with my own mind, education and knowledge. I began to realize the way I thought or perceived things was always related to food in my mind. It takes around thirty days to change a habit they say. Is it possible then gaining weight is a bunch of bad habits and bad choices, perhaps that could be true I wondered?

Game changing is a term we have all heard but I do not really like that term. Maybe if weight was a game, however it is no game. Weight is about me and it is about you and it involves feelings of having to be uncomfortable or downright miserable or ashamed with how you look or feel and that is no game, certainly no game anyone wishes to engage in voluntarily. Onward to a better healthier way of weight now though. You should now think those old feelings are just no longer acceptable and you do not wish to allow them to be part of your life any longer.

THE A-HA MOMENT

ॐ

> *"Now for the good news. I experienced my weight loss A-ha moment using Full Belly Meter System and I believe you can benefit too using my really simple system."*

The Full Belly Meter © weight loss system is a very special reading experience for all fellow weight wrenched hearts who have spent countless months; years and even entire lives struggling with their weight. People place great importance on A-ha moments because this is when we gain awareness to something we did not realize before and this creates the moment of essential clarity that we were missing. We also gain insight to patterns we have in our lives and insight into our own behaviors when the moment of essential clarity presents itself.

" I WANT MY A-HA MOMENT "

"That is what I used to say to myself all of the time. I was unhappy for years as you may be now. I am not unhappy any longer and found my moment. I want to show you and teach you how I arrived at my moment and how the suggested system works.

Finally, being shown something important you never knew about or realized for your own default body food and mind system interaction could be just what you have been searching for."

I have learned from my journey that to achieve this clarity to the point where it becomes the default operating system of my body and not just making a short modification to the outcome, that the insight to the clarity has to be applied to get there because you will not just transform like magic just like that. Think of going somewhere, for example from your home to the grocery store.

You do not just think it and then you are there. You actually need to step or walk or run or do something to get there. There is something that you do extra in between the two points that gets you from point A to point B which is your destination. I recall always wondering before where my personal A-ha moment was. I could not put my finger on it - but just knew something was missing somewhere. It felt like so many pieces of the puzzle were present – for example, all of the wonderfully delicious low calorie meals, super low calorie nutritious cookbooks, slow cooker dinners, even lower calorie cookies, candies and snacks. It was all in the books and on the internet and anywhere you can find that should have just taken me there – to my A-ha moment but sadly, never did. I recall thinking hmmm - there seemed to be something askew, something not right with all that information available and to not achieve my A-ha moment. There are a few missing pieces but what were they I kept asking myself over through those beginning years. I would question what some others seem to have figured out when I would look at the success stories on YouTube. I would wonder how these other success stories I saw getting to their goals were doing afterward on maintaining and in general and I learned that 90% of them would be putting that weight back on after 1 to 2 years which just seemed like a waste of time effort and money to me.

More and more it was apparent I had to get healthy to lose the weight and have a repeatable cognitive correcting braintrain system to establish that brain to body connection until it became more automatic, more default in order to help change my bad food and bad human habits.

I also found studies that people who keep food diaries are proven to lose TWICE – YES TWICE AS MUCH weight as those who do not – hence the workbook at the end of this book!

With The Full Belly Meter System it is more likely for you to become the master of yourself, to get more control and this suggested system truly makes you so unbelievably accountable to yourself that you will be amazed and surprised at yourself and your journey.

If you can turn your weight around like I did, even if it is a bit at a time, then I have succeeded in conveying properly to you in paying it forward to you with my suggested system. Fast weight loss is not always the best answer nor is it always optimally healthy. My personal belief is that 1-2 pounds a week done the whole healthy system lifestyle way is optimal and will help last toward that much longer haul. Join us at **www.fullbellymeter.com** and also join our thriving free facebook weightloss support group at #theweightlossboss with Katherine Giesbrecht that offers you 24/7 – 365 weightloss daily motivational, inspirational and educational support.

STRAIGHT UP IN YOUR FACE

&

"Don't Complicate It"

> *Let's think out of the box together – what if there is nothing wrong with you or your thinking?*
>
> *What if all you needed was some good old straightforward, simple mind food education with my easiest straight forward common sense system – The Full Belly Meter © System.*

So - simply - straight up – in your face – for you, is this information and my system. Don't complicate it because it truly is not a complicated system to learn, in fact it is so easy and straight forward that it becomes fun to do and not a chore.

Even with my medical condition hurdles, the kind that seem to stop most weight loss in its tracks for people; it was still easy to overcome these issues using my system because getting healthy was key. The biggest nutritional bang for my buck plus using the system to me was superior.

For my whole life I had always thought that a weight loss method, plan or system has to be pretty complicated and have a ton of documentation or something complex behind it to work. Given my earlier adolescence thinking that eating something that would create a calorie deficit in my cells just had to work and must be something that needs a ton of proven research and if there was research to say so then it must just work right? In reality, contrary to that, I am here to tell you that no, there is other weight related factors. There needs to be sufficient proper protein intake to create satiety that lasts, plus good fats, the good carbs and less of the bad carbs, hidden sugars and in your face sugars that have to go and fat free items but also fat-free labels that will fool you and things that are nice and weight loss causing that have little nutrition in them!

I became acutely aware that to understand weight loss involves calories yes which are a 'unit of food energy' but next I would need to know what type of food energy and what else aside from that my body required to remain full and not be hungry (satiety) but still create the deficit. This involved maximizing protein to what my body needed, plus nutrient rich choices of foods and macronutrients and getting healthy plus lifestyle changes. I also realized that food is extremely personal plus individual and that one food or recipe will not work the same for another.

My friend could whip up a wonderful recipe and eat lots of something and loose or maintain her weight with it. However, if I ate that exact same thing I never got the same results. Thanks to individual DNA, family histories, aging and metabolisms, different ethnic cultural backgrounds, and medical conditions and more it only makes sense that what worked for her may not work for me to the same degree. I wanted to take that whole kit and caboodle process out of the box put it on paper for you in a short easy to begin, easy to follow sample format.

A novice can just jump in and start right away if they wish. By now you are probably wondering if The Full Belly Meter © System involves any kind of super intense work, writing or tracking or calorie counting at all. I am telling you yes absolutely! it is essential to track because studies prove those who do lose TWO times the amount, TWICE as much weight as those who do not. This is so simple to learn and once your connection happens the body defaults to that connection which helps keeps you constantly accountable. Yes of course you will have to put in some initial work same as I did to start in order to work towards your destination.   However, to be able to drop a lot of that work load after that to a much lower level or hopefully drop the work load altogether like I pretty much do to this day is to me just the best system ever.   I rarely still need to count, track or write anything down or do any of those things on a daily basis and I can still continue to go down on my scale when I want to. The type of happiness I was seeking has arrived at last I can say.   Put in your faith to give it 30 to get sturdy!   That first 30 days is learning 'the bridge' then you redefine and finetune as you go forward.   Just put in a little effort to gain your reward – I promise you that you will thank yourself for the small amount of work required from you.

YES, YOU CAN STILL HAVE SUCCESS WITH NO EXERCISE

ॐ

#fullbellymeter

When I looked around at successful stories or popular programs while developing my personal system I noticed an emphasis was always being put on exercising or getting a lot of activity in but I had a personal problem! I had to ask myself how I was going to do that when I had one of my arthritic pain days and exercise just wasn't possible. Or how about when I was having a bad thyroid day and exercising was possible but I had to work 10 times harder than the person in the video I was watching to get the same results because my thyroid just did not want to work normally. I recall thinking to myself, how long in my lifetime will I be physically able to exercise for life and keep this all up. It became evidently clear to me that as time moves forward, my body will not move forward and I won't be able to twist around like a prima donna nor stand any type of real impact any much longer. I knew I had a challenge coming up and had to think logically through it to lose the weight without the exercise. I jotted this down in my notebook and starred it saying, 'no exercise'. I had no idea how to find a way to get there with this thought in mind but I thought write it down anyways, address it later. I loved exercise when I was younger and I would say flat out it really does help bring those inches in tighter and make you feel better and help your health overall by exercising and it will burn calories; improve my cardiovascular, help build lean muscle, burn that fat and many other benefits. The thing I needed for myself and want all readers to realize is I suspect there is a very big portion of us out there that cannot at times hit the gyms or the floors like the others and may have to get a handle on just the food and negative behaviors first. We are all unique on how we are going to get there. All I am simply getting at is that my system will still help you towards success if you are like I was for a period of time; and at that point in time just could not get or keep that exercise or activity into my daily routine right from the start.   I was only doing my usual activity in later life for example getting up in the morning, walking to the kitchen to make my coffee, turning on the television and so on so I think you get the picture now. That is all forms of activity but it is natural day to day activity my body is already used to.

TIP !

If you want to have some fun list every piece of exercise equipment you purchased and what you spent on it. Then compare that to the cost of this book and system. I did this myself and was amazed to realize just how much money I spent on machines. They did help me when I could use them but they never were the sole solution that gave me my 'A-ha' moment for more permanent healthy weight loss.

CHAPTER 2

START DAY REALLY MATTERS

ℬ

True or not true? Normally start day does matter. What day you choose to start your journey will matter on most systems or plans.

To move ahead at maximum speed on Full Belly Meter just start right away no matter the day. On other systems it is usually better to start on a Monday. Most diets, plans and systems get you to start eating their suggestions right away so if you start on the day of a weekend wedding or that weekend of getting together with your friends then you are bound to make it tougher for yourself. With other systems you may not want to begin right away and have to wait for the Monday.

However, with the Full Belly Meter © system, it actually will not matter what day you start and here is why.

"Start on any day you wish because for the first suggested 3 days you remain eating what you have always been eating. So if you start on a weekend, a holiday, wedding or birthday then it will not matter."

That is another wonderful thing to know about this awesome system is that you can get started the minute you pick up the book and get going any day you please. There is no need to wait for the wedding, the birthday or the Valentines dinner or Christmas party, just get started.

If you are a person like me, impatient when it comes to getting the weight off then flip to Chapter 4's section called 'The Full Belly System Quick Step Start List' and get going. Then come back and finish reading the rest of the book.

The system book here remember is just 'The Bridge' the BadAss Belly Braintrain to help create a newer better behavior – the book is your basic steps and bridge to learn insight on how to get your belly to brain connection established. Also visit our website and free facebook group to see more if you want to do the full circle and learn to benefit moreso by doing the fuller healthier nutrition-bang for buck packed way. Visit our website for more advanced suggestions in courses and video's plus we have links to our free weightloss support group where someone is always there to support you.

GETTING STARTED

&

First and always is said to check with your doctor before trying Full Belly System © or any food suggestion or modification, diet or system to make sure it is ok for you. Gastric surgery patients, any weight related surgery patients, pregnant persons, under legal age, any Prader Willie Syndrome Patients need specialized care and to be under the guidance of your doctors! Do not follow this system in these situations so people with any medical conditions need to use your Doctors recommended food dietary instructions. This is important because you may have medical conditions or situations that he or she may feel requires a different approach or path that is best for you. That will be left up to you and your doctor to decide for yourselves and if you proceed ahead with any information from this book it is of your own free will and doing and you agree to move forward at your own expense and own consequences. Always better safe than sorry I say and because I am the type of author that actually cares about you getting to your goals safely and soundly I really do believe it is in your best interest to clear any plan you try including this system with your doctor. Now with all that being said and if you have your physician clearance and you are ready to begin then we can get started. There is no need to study up, read long reports, put together complicated systems or dig for information to get started. Just read my book and about the system, highlight anything of importance to you that you think you should remember as key, and then begin the workbook pages at the back of this book. In no time at all if you are diligent at this to start, exciting things may happen in your life like happened in mine. It is just so easy to begin. First thing to know is that you will be doing all of your initial grunt work and recording in the workbook section included with this book. That is where all of your DIY magic truly begins so refer to the chapter workbook section at the end of the book. Remember that recording is the groundwork or hard work as I call it to get to your easier way of life with none to very little recording later on – the recording should be temporary and not forever needed which is such a nice change and one of my own personal goals that I had really hoped to accomplish when I set out on my own journey. You will step on that scale in the morning when you get up and record your morning weight in the top left corner of the workbook pages for at least the next thirty days. Remember you are the boss of your system and I only suggest 30 days but one can do more say sixty, ninety days or whatever length you choose but thirty days is what I did for myself and my brain got it, so whatever it takes for you is what it is.

TIP !

For those sticklers who really want to know their exact progress step on the scale a second time around after you are dressed in the morning. Your clothes add weight so you will know in your mind eventually where you stand in any scenario and how much that clothing really is adding to your scale. You would be surprised probably at just how much weight a pair of jeans, shirt, socks, belt and shoes can add to that scale. Next, it is suggested to plan to record your night weight located in the workbook down at the bottom right corner of your workbook right before bed that same night and every night thereafter for at least the next thirty days. REMEMBER 30 TO GET STURDY!

Repeat this process morning and night faithfully. My night time weight is usually two to four pounds heavier for myself than my morning weight and yours may vary some as well but do not fear that you are screwing it up if you see a pretty big gain between your morning and evening numbers. That is natural I have learned by just recording my own data for a period of time and is how my own body behaves. By repeating recording morning and night you will be taking personal inventory of how your body is behaving and reacting. The recording is suggested to be done morning and night because everyone is not the same when it comes to the weight up or down daily amount. You may be a person who goes up and down by one pound per day or by five even up to seven pounds within that time frame I have heard of. The only way you can know how your body behaves is to put in the initial work and start recording. It really forces you to pay attention to what your body registers once you have finished consuming for that day. Just one really important thing – the weighing in is not something I had to do forever for my own success thank goodness to that. This was such another super bonus to my system I discovered from my own experience. The weighing in morning and night in the beginning however is important for the destination steps to clarity. The more whole clarity you achieve, the less you need to weigh in but then again that is going to need to be up to you as to when you wish to stop the daily recording. You will stop recording when you achieve clarity just automatically. Remember this is going to be your baby, your DIY project on yourself so to speak and my experience and success is just your suggested guideline to help you get to your goals and make your life easier like mine has become. At the least do enough recording of days in a row to get to the point where if you find you miss a day, then two or three days' recordings and then a week at a time or more but you find you are still losing the weight – that is your happy signal to your brain that you as well are onto the A-ha moment path via the Full Belly Meter © system and well onto a happier you. No one wants to have to record forever. Recording macronutrients, numbers or food items, perhaps calories, carbs, activities or whatever it may be can become so very tedious and a downright chore. Certainly I just did not see myself being the only one that felt that way inside and wanted to see if I could somehow tweak my system to make things easier than that. So I recall I kept pushing forward, the more I stuck to it the more the clarity came through and the easier it truly became. I felt motivation from others going through what I was experiencing was important and as well to be able to do the rest at home on my own and still succeed – I felt that would be ideal for me and same for you so we also have for you to join free our support group (visit our website). I can tell you by doing Full Belly Meter ©

for a short period of time, I was working toward my personal goals and achieving them with less and less effort in a really truly acceptable time frame than ever before in my whole life. By morning and nightly weighing in, this taught how the body responded scale wise to the foods put in it every twelve to twenty-four hours. This is actually a vital brain step and something you to know and to embrace fully and repeatedly in the beginning but not forever. The information becomes very valuable to you and to your clarity later on. It is also really neat to be able to flip through the left top or bottom right workbook pages like an old fashioned movie put together frame by frame and see your numbers change like a movie when you have enough days recorded to flip through. It is inspiring. I personally feel a more successful weight loss system cannot just present a blanket food item list and recipe book to follow. What I mean by that is to get everyone to eat the same foods and expect to get the exact same results is just ludicrous to me. I do not believe that is the best A-ha path or way to the desired more permanent personal and individual weight loss solution when you try to eat what everyone else is. If you can eat what you really like or eat what you are accustomed to and belly that up, you are way more likely to end up loving this and not feeling guilty either about what you are eating. I recall being at work discussing weight loss with a coworker. She was talking about a revamped plan that was launched and how she did not think it could work for her. She said to me quote "Don't take this the wrong way but you white people eat different". Her comment intrigued me and it made sense to me why she felt that way and that the plan she was looking at may not work very well for her. I thought to myself later on this is why Full Belly Meter also becomes even more wonderful because anyone can do it from anywhere and they are in control of it and not someone else. Anyone can do this I thought.

When you start the suggested workbook section aside from your weight recording you will be recording what is going into your body as well on a daily basis for the next at least thirty, sixty to ninety days at least. Remember this is the DIY part where you do whatever it takes for your body to brain mind connection to achieve clarity. For food recording, you start day one through day three of your Full Belly workbook section with what you normally eat on a daily basis, do not diet, scrimp or change your normal intake and just write down what you eat and be honest about it. So to be more explanatory do not calorie down any items or eat sparingly, just eat whatever you have been regularly eating on a daily normal basis and then take that to the stuffed meter feeling level and record it all down, include drinks and snacks – everything that went into the mouth until you could feel your stomach stuffed (but not in pain). So your first three days of workbook entries should look like this. Day 1 shows date, morning weigh in amount, list of all items consumed, record when you hit the just stuffed feeling and finally your night time weight. Do it again – repeat daily to at least day three. 3 days of reaching stuffed is enough, then stop going to stuffed. My goal when I started was to survive on my own. What I mean is I was trying to get to where I could handle this on my own, without meetings, without books to follow, without pills to take or exercise machines to use. I just thought to myself it would be so nice to just survive on my own without all the frills and whistles, just to one day wake up and be healthier and happier and thinner without all of the fuss. I would just sit and think about maintaining my weight loss on my own and eventually staying that way. Once the mind body food connection gets combined to your daily pen paper and weight numbers it starts becoming 'one'. The A-ha moment is getting closer. So you choose when you feel you got the hang of recording eating normally what you eat to the point of realizing when you feel stuffed – then you stop and write it all down. The stuffed feeling, what time it happened, what you ate and any emotions with that i.e.: sad that you ate all that cake and pizza or sad you ate every bag of chips around you as you know it cannot be helping your image in the mirror. It is not recommended to continue eating to 'stuffed' after your first 3 days, and you have documented that for yourself. Normally it takes only 3 days to achieve insight for what the scale says to what you did for that day for your normal daily intake as recall even though you eat your regular routine for 3 days you are documenting your weight morning and night. Next move on to now defining your plan for yourself and continue recording daily as you go.

STUFFED FULL HERE WE GO

೮౨

Plan to temporarily feel just stuffed (recall the suggested 3 days or whatever amount of days is needed to make that braintrain cognitive behavior connection) however a few days should do it. Food wise I recall in the beginning my thoughts were that I really need to plan to stuff myself until my belly said that it could not take another bite. I

> *"Plan To Temporarily Really Feel Stuffed Suggested Is A Few Days; But Not Make Yourself Sick In Doing So".*
>
> *By using the right items individual to yourself as explained in Full Belly Meter, eventually your scale just may make you want to smile like you have not done in a very long time.*

still to this day do not know why I did that. I just thought what the heck; I have been holding myself back for over twenty years trying portion control to everything else and I was already screwed blued and tattooed as nothing was getting through permanently. Since that never really got me where I wanted to be I wanted to push myself and my thinking out of the box and out of my normal comfort zone. If I gained ten more pounds from my experiment then what the heck, I am already suffering I figured so why not have to give a little to get something is what I thought in my mind. What I got was a surprise. I did not get a huge rise in the scale because I started with what I always ate anyways and obviously I was eating a lot because it did not take that much more to hit the just stuffed feeling. So recall that suggested is for day one through day three; plan to eat what you normally eat and just record your morning and nightly weight in your workbook section and all of what you ate till you recognize level 2 or 3. If you wish to track any other system or method you are already used to counting then go right ahead alongside this. I have included spots for that in the workbook at the back of this book for you to do that if you wish as there is no need to drop what you already know because it will just aid you forward till you do not need it anymore. When I began my journey, in forefront in my mind the thought kept occurring to eat to be just stuffed (temporarily of course, not for a long period nor forever). Just enough so I could begin to recognize the brain to belly connection faster and faster. I ate so much so that until my belly meter measured fully stuffed is when I would stop and have to break away from the routine foods I would eat. I did this for the first few days. You choose how long you wish to do this for, I did this as I said for a few days myself then moved on to my next steps but you are your own boss with this system and you use your own schedule that works for you. That is the beauty of this system in that it becomes tailored just for you – made by you, followed by you, detailed for you – by you and I just teach you the steps on how to bridge that belly to brain connection. Realize that the overall goal of my eating what I always ate for the first few days till I was just stuffed had a real purpose, this was to train my brain to realize that trigger feeling, the full belly meter signal and get used to that stuffed signal from belly to brain. It is a very important and key feature of Full Belly Meter to know and be able to recognize that feeling and document it when it hits. I trained my brains thoughts to really shout at me. Like it is speaking to you and inside your head it says I am just stuffed or your thoughts say I just have to put down this fork or I just could not eat another bite. That sort of conveyance is what I am talking about. That is all about learning and experiencing the feelings for the Full Belly Meter feeling. At that point your meter would be registering on just stuffed and mission is accomplished on that one belly to brain signal learning suggested task. Next on these beginning days keep in mind that included in my goal was to push myself and see what it was like to stay belly stuffed or stuffed 'all day long' and not just for an hour or so. The point was to achieve a steady flow of feeling no hunger. Incorporating sufficient protein for satiety, and adding my other nutrition packed macronutrients was vital, so my body did not crave for any foods and to stay feeling satisfied and stuffed. I wanted to achieve feeling full and happy and not wanting for food. I did not want however to be overstuffed to the point where I felt sick as then I would have overdone it. I worked toward being able to finally just bypass food joints or places or items that trigger massive cravings calling out my name. You probably think I am joking but it is for real, if you are satiated; and cannot eat anymore then you actually can bypass all of those places now because your stomach and mind is so full you just do not want that item at that time. HAL-E-LUYAH !!! When you notice you can drive by those places loaded with fat and calories and sugar that normally call your name and you just keep going you are well on your way to mastering the Full Belly Meter System Bridge (The BadAss Belly Braintrain). Furthermore, to mastering this part, another goal is to be able to drive by that food joint that you can smell; or walk by it and still be content even though you smell is wafting by you – calling out your name. To be not craving no matter the signage flashing at you, the visual piece of food you see going by or the smells emanating by or around you is part of what I really feel is an important piece to achieving a longer term successful journey. It becomes a marker of personal cognitive success for yourself when you can do this and you will realize it very quickly when it begins to happen. Believe it or not, it was really possible for me to eventually accomplish this on the Full Belly Meter system. This may sound sort of crazy at this time to you; but is really not crazy at all. This is because the more I achieved being able to drive by, walk by and just keep going on smells, lights and signs while being just stuffed from the right things for my body then the closer I got to the ultimate a-ha path or achieving clarity. Ongoing with Full Belly Meter System © I finally came to realize that prior to my system when doing any plan or system with something else I had been always reaching for snacks or in-betweens because I was just not satiated, in other words I still had room to fill the bucket up some more and because I could, I sure would. The more evenly satiated I stayed throughout my day just in the beginning; then the less snacking or wanting for chips, crackers, cakes and cookies I felt. My scale proved this to me as well. This was another nice surprise on my new journey that I was not expecting but nonetheless a very welcome discovery indeed. Really important is the inner belly voice or belly thoughts to rise through to the mind and alert the brain that the belly is just stuffed and cannot take another piece of food – the signal. By now I realized that is just so important to know and recognize to succeed with my system. The 'Belly Braintrain' is what I called it at first, by logging or recording in the workbook section for two times daily, writing down every morsel you are put in the mouth and eating to maintain being just stuffed for those beginning days helped my body go through the motions to the natural A-ha or clarity boot camp steps as I call it. So just remember then to start there is no need to calorie it down or anything like that in those first few days. Just write down what you normally eat and if you are like me in the beginning and you want to compare later on your calories, macronutrients, carbs or any counting system you currently use or are used to. There are fields in the workbook section provided for you that you can enter whatever you wish to count or want to keep track of. I learned at the end of my trial notebook I carried around with me that in as little as thirty days that I need not do this forever. I also learned from my data that I wrote down that it would help me later on to find equal or better tasting belly find healthier nutrition packed replacements that really worked with Full Belly System © to create my calorie deficit goal but leave me really satisfied. So although not required in the beginning to count calories, I did for the first month and I found it helped me go back and belly my stuff up later on so I would suggest try at least for the first month to record all of the calories associated with what you took in, record everything food and drink, emotions, exercise, vitamins and your scaling. Remember people who record lose TWICE as much weight in past studies done.

In order for my mind to get that just stuffed message from my full belly meter to my brain it only took a few days and not much extra food and I was ready to ride the braintrain after that. With my full belly meter signals working full blow to my brain I was ready to take this to my next level.

FULL BELLY METER LEVELS

ℬ

The Full Belly Meter © scale is simplified to be only three levels to keep track of or be able to sense in the mind. This is important and works toward the brain belly body train. The A-ha recognition moment.

1) Hungry
2) Full
3) Just Stuffed (but not sick)

When starting out I sought option 3 as much as possible as it was optimal to me learning about my belly and my thoughts connecting to the food I ate. I stuck to option 3 until my body was tired of being so stuffed but really 3 days of that and I 'got it'. Eventually my body on its own started backing down on the amount of food I required to get this feeling as it just naturally begins and my body naturally was ready to take it down a few notches on its own. I definitely noticed I required less amount of food over time to feel satisfied while my stomach shrank. This of course was not just due to eating a bunch of food, I was constantly revamping my bad habits and bad choices as well to become as nutritional as possible and do what I could to become healthier.

CHAPTER 3

☙

ATTENDING THE SCHOOL OF SELFIE

"Photos and a pair of shorts with string in the waist"

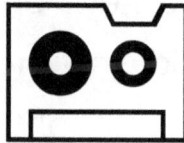

Grab a selfie or current photo of yourself. If you can, take one or several front views and one or several side views. Put them away for later.

You may not like your photograph being taken at this point however it is nice to have it later on for personal viewing and for personal comparison purposes.

I would suggest a fully clothed full body photo or two and some head shots from front and side. It is pretty surprising to realize how a 15 lb weight loss can show up on your face or on your body. I saw a neat YouTube video one time of a person who snapped her photo every 15 pounds consistently. It was an eye opener because even at 15 pounds I could see the transformation so that was pretty cool I thought. Also considering I was used to the old-fashioned thinking of taking a photo when you start and when you reach your destination you may want to change it up in one fashion or another when it comes to your selfies.

Next grab a pair of shorts or sweats that have a draw string that you tie up in the front. A cheapie pair will do that you can use for your personal physical and visual reminder of where you have been and where you are.

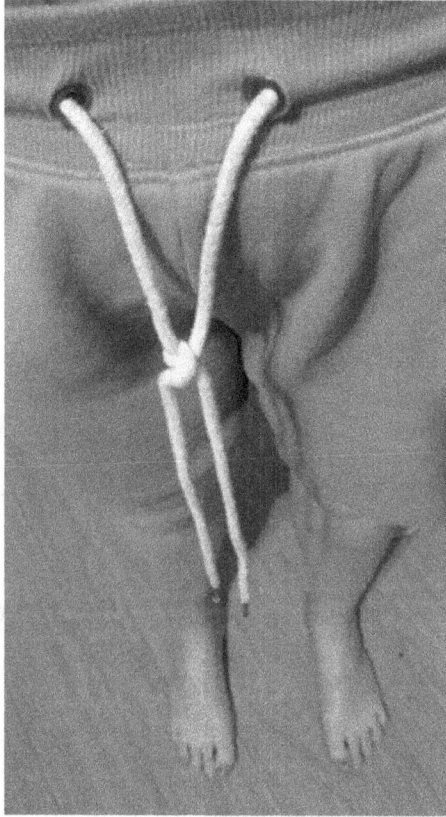

Above you see my own personal pair of shorts I use. This pair of shorts or sweats is intended to replace any daily tape measuring as it is good to change it up and see real clothing progress – the loose string becoming longer and longer - verses numbers on a tape measure.

Stick the shorts or sweats in your drawer for later use and reference. I pull mine out about every 3 weeks or so and put them on. This has become something I look forward to doing now as it is always a positive for me.

Drawstring Instructions:

Put on your drawstring shorts or sweats. For myself I personally use a pair of soft shorts with a drawstring. Then next draw the string comfortable at your waist, not too tight, not too loose keeping it just right with a relaxed stomach. If the fit feels just right and comfortable tie the string in that exact spot. Tie it crazy solid so it never comes undone again just like mine. Make it a solid knot that cannot get undone in the washing machine or what have you. Make sure it is nice and solid and undoable. You should not need to undo this string ever again if your mind has made the A-ha connection. These shorts become your personal measuring tool, replacing your tape measure method. As often as you wish, you will be throwing on these shorts or sweats as you move forward on your personal journey.

At first you will begin to realize there is some play in your string. Then you will notice it is starting to hang looser. Then you will notice your string hangs and hangs more and more.

My string hangs down about 4 to 5 inches on each side as you can see in my photo which means without a measuring tape I can physically really see the impact that is occurring to my body.

Right now, I love those old ugly shorts when I throw them on, they have elastic in the waist with the string in the waist band so still stay on. Without a tape measure, that string really brings me into focus. I find it just amazing and it gives me my mind check back to stark reality of something I can really see instead of numbers on the tape. The reality of where I came from to where I am is startling and personally satisfying when seeing that string. I am going to save those old shorts forever in a drawer – they are my reality check and I think you will love this method for yourself to because it is just fun, raises awareness to self and rewarding to self.

🎁 T I P !

For those numbers people you can still record your tape measure numbers, if that works for you then go for it. Or if you forget to use your tape measure and really wanted to know what you were in the start, just measure the amount of loose string on your shorts to figure out your numbers in inches. If you wish to record any tape measurements right now for later reference you can do that too below:

Measurements for Date: _____

Chest: _____

Arms: _____

Waist: _____

Hips: _____

Legs: _____

Other: _____

GET ARMED WITH YOUR TOOLKIT

ༀ

1) Your selfie photos
2) Your drawstring shorts or sweats
3) Digital scale
4) Internet Access and YouTube if you have
5) Kitchen tools or gadgets for easier progress
6) Support groups, chats etc.

Selfie Photos:

Glue them into this book or put them in your drawer. Decide in your mind at what amount of weight loss you will be doing for your next selfie's. A nice suggested guideline is incremented goals of 5-10% of your total weight. You are the boss, so you decide but write down on the back of your selfie or print out the date and weight you are at each time you do a new one. You would be amazed if you even compare a 15 lb loss in a photo as it can really reshape a face.

Drawstring shorts or sweats:
Keep them handy to throw on whenever, over time you'll get that quick visual omg somethings changing reminder.

Digital Scale (is a must have item):
I like a digital scale because I can see my weight change in ounces and believe me all of them count. Did you know a smaller tube of toothpaste is 2 to 4 ounces and a larger one is 6.5 ounces on average so if you have gone down 6 ounces that is actually very positive. Just think you lost the equivalent to a regular size tube of toothpaste. Put that in your hand and you can really feel the weight.

YouTube: Never underestimate the power of internet, YouTube and weight loss assistance. I have looked up countless information on tips and tricks and inspirational videos for weight loss. I cannot say enough about how wonderful and helpful these can be. There is also free in-home walking exercise videos and many more exciting things to watch.

Kitchen Tools:

Kitchen tools are an ongoing lifetime investment. For example, I picked up a multi-cooker machine with a paddle in it that uses just one tablespoon of oil and boy the grilled garlic shrimp or home made fries come out fantastically tasting with a tablespoon of my ghee butter I use; or some coconut oil. I also picked up a potato electric mashing tool and that has really taken the chore out of mashing my potatoes. Whatever makes your life easier in the kitchen is going to be good for you and your journey. Investing in your kitchen and yourself is highly recommended.

Support Groups, Classes, Chats Etc.:

Support in weightloss is essential, it is KEY to staying on track and getting motivation and inspirations. Without it, you are more likely to fail.

You will be with likeminded people at our Facebook group; where you can share your thoughts, successes, bumbles, and is just great because we are there 24/7 – 365 and put out every single day a motivation or inspiration to keep you on track – WELL WORTH THE FREE JOIN!

A support system never hurts and is always going to be to your better benefit and final goal I feel.

To join our free support group just visit www.fullbellymeter.com for more information.

COMFORT FOODS ARE KEYS WITH LOCKS ON THEM

ॐ

"Comfort foods and eating in moderation defined"

EATING IN MODERATION

Learning about how your body responds on your scale to the foods you consume can tell you so much more than you realize. The foods you consume all the time, some of the ones you absolutely love and eat over and over can actually become a few keys to happiness instead of your sadness when changed up in a personal way.

Have you heard that saying "If it is not on your fork, it is in your mouth" well then what if it was a good thing. It sounds weird to think that when on a weight loss journey but ultimately you want it this to be a good thing – a good feeling. Eating in moderation or portion control alone is not enough but you do need to learn a key for long term weight loss which is to not 'overeat'.

But for starting the Braintrain suggested first 3 days, eating moderately will not trigger the full belly meter feeling properly. Recall earlier I spoke of not craving and not being hungry (changing my bad cognitive food behavior).

The mind needs to be taught about real comfort food – satiating nutrient packed – and enough of it in the beginning to not be starving hungry & have sufficient protein, good carbs and good fats and you feel energized.   In turn you should be happy, full and best of all down on the scale if you have mastered the Full Belly Meter System © like I did.

COMFORT ZONE

ଚ୨

In my early days of developing my system, with pen and paper in hand, day by day – the thoughts kept rolling in and I would just keep jotting them down until I saw or developed anything for my bad patterns (bad cognitive behaviors), any idea or anything that may make some sense later on when looking back at it all. I gained realization when looking back at my daily lists that I was a real true creature of habit always heading to my favorite go-to foods and I had this really small list of things I just wanted again and again and would eat pretty much the same thing over and over.

So I began to wonder, what if I could make a few of those favorite negatives into favorite positives for myself – this could be key for me.

COMFORT FOODS IN DEPTH

COMFORT IS KEY

ॐ

Comfort foods for the purpose of my system will be extremely personal to you and extremely important to you. You will write down your current comfort foods list and number them in order by importance. You can start right at home right away. If you are not sure where to begin your list open your fridge, cupboards, pantry or freezer. Start writing down everything you would normally grab to eat for yourself. Just jot down the favorites you normally pick first. After you are done with that add any restaurant or drive thru items outside of the home that are your favorites as well. Do not worry about how long your list is, it will not matter the length or how many items are on it.

Once finished your list itemize it by order of importance to yourself. This becomes truly personal to you and key to your goals and success. For example, my own number one comfort food has probably got to be pizza. That went on the top of my list because I ate it often and love it and eat way more than just one slice.

So your most often eaten favorite food will be number one on your list and so on till you have numbered your whole list. Be sure to include all go-to food or beverage, sauces, snacks or desserts that you consistently love and eat as it all counts towards you gaining success. A future goal is that some of your personal list will become the very keys to unlocking your weight over time in a positive way rather than a negative way. You should not have to completely give up all comfort foods on your list; as you will find something that works better on your scales numbers but that sugar, bad fats and bad carbs will just need to go.

** Belly Up **. In the dictionary it says to go belly up means a fail. There is another description in the dictionary that refers to a dead animal on the roadside belly up, yuck that sounded just so terrible when I read that one but it made me realize it can be a fail – a big fail. If one of your go-to comfort foods makes your scale rise it has gone belly up and FAILED. It is simply a failed recipe or failed food energy source which means it can be modified in one way or another to become a more successful comfort food for you.

COMFORT SHOULD FEEL LIKE THIS

℘

When you feel comfort from a comfort food it should look something like this on the Full Belly System. The fat should come off your plate so that your body pulls the fat from your belly instead; you should be satiated with healthy food choices, the scales numbers should be going downward, you can know from your workbook entries that the things you love and consumed affected your weight in a positive fashion and it was delicious to eat. Picture feeling full, satisfied and healthy as each day goes by and those numbers keep decreasing clothes become looser, and things like bending over start getting easier and all from foods you now love and were able to adjust even a few comfort ones to be really healthy comfort foods instead of negative stress foods. Then you can know you have truly found a comfort food that is working for you. To recap that a little differently you should be able to know that you ate something that was very tasty to you and that you were able to feel full and satisfied for long periods; and you were able to smile when you stepped on that scale.

BRAIN CHANGING

೮೦

Once you develop your comfort foods list – refer back to that list and expand and improve on it always – never give up, always look for ways to improve it and try new things. You may have changes in your top favorites over time so adjust your list and minus or add things eventually as well.

The comfort foods are the ones that make you want to reach for them, to FEEL COMFORTABLE IN HEART MIND, SOUL ** AND ON THE SCALE!** You have to feel comfort on the scale to succeed – it cannot be just comfort in the mind only or belly only when you do the system. A lot of people have been groomed by society to think that comfort foods can only be the crappy calorie fat carb saturated foods. That sort of thinking can be turned around if you know how to change your brain and your ingredients.

After you pigged out and ate your regular daily routine of foods; maybe a few thousand calories worth or more and your scale goes up in numbers then that is the moment standing in the nature on your scale (why wear clothes when standing on it as it means more weight) to realize that what you ate was not 'comfortable' at all. In fact, looking at the numbers increasing – you actually feel downright miserable and very uncomfortable. Recognize that miserableness for what it truly is.

It is ** NOT COMFORT to be miserable **. Hence your comfort food did not comfort you at all !

So seriously we are all told we are gluttons for our comfort foods and that is why we are fat or at least a lot of us write fat off in our minds thinking like this. I know I used to think like this all the time.

So, what would happen if you ate comfort foods that reversed your numbers on the scale downwards and made you feel very comfortable standing there looking at those numbers. That would be a really awesome feeling – and you can do it, you can achieve this.

Try to visualize or recall the feelings of that moment when you stepped on the scale and your weight rose, or you looked in the mirror and did not like the weight or what you saw as you tried to button up a nice shirt and it was not possible. Or say that the buttons were pulling apart ridiculously and you felt like you looked stupid, or you tried to buckle up those pants and you could not and you felt just utterly defeated by your own fat. ** That is NOT COMFORT **

Or recall perhaps when you wanted to cross your legs and you could not. You could not even raise your leg high enough to try and cross them or you could just cross your ankles only and not swing one leg over the other like your co-worker or your friend or someone else you saw and watched in envy. Or how about when someone wanted to hug you but you did not let them because you felt ashamed and just too fat to receive that love. They never knew this, they just thought you did not want their affection or maybe thought you were just a cold person and that really was not the case at all. You were just not comfortable is what it really was.

Or recall the time you wanted to go for family photos but did not because you felt too big – or how about when you wanted to put on a bathing suit, or a bikini and did not.

How about the time you received a beautiful piece of jewelry and you put it on horrified that it did not hang on your neck properly and was more like a choker than a showpiece, or it did not fit your wrist or ankle like it should have. Maybe you could not even do it up because you were just too big.

The point of me bringing this to light is YOU ARE NOT ALONE and many other people feel and experience the same things you do and they do not like it either. It is not comfortable at all and is life damaging to have to go through any of that I felt personally. You should be getting the picture by now of what I am getting at which the topic is comfort. Question yourself, ask your mind to be honest with yourself and see if you can relate to even one or all of the above scenarios.

Can you really authenticate to your mind after thinking about this; that your comfort foods you have been consuming prior to this suggested Full

Belly Meter Weight Loss system were truly giving you honest comfortable feelings. You need to make the connection that you did not truly consume comfort foods because when the results are not desirable and staring, no – glaring at you in your face and you do not like the feeling then you know your comfort food is A BROKEN FOOD.

You will need your broken foods to be bellied up - properly, maximize your bang for your nutrition-buck.

NOW – Picture having a week or two of being into your workbook, picture having some success with your numbers and imagine what a few more weeks or months might do. Then imagine what would happen if you made it to that 30-day habit changing range or you make it to clarity. Picture your comfort food list growing and you just eating delicious stuff that you love and do not need to force yourself to eat. Picture going to the fridge and not having to calculate and plan about really what you are grabbing; but that you have stocked and planned your fridge and your life with the right things so whatever you grab will produce comfort to you. Picture that you feel comfort with what you ate. Imagine you felt comfortable getting on and off the scale and the whole time you were just stuffed and loving it all.

What will you think when the numbers on the scale start to reverse for the good and the numbers start telling you your personal story in black and white.

Telling you what you are doing right and what you have been doing wrong and what you can improve on. To me that is a cool thing, to be able to get positive numbers from doing this on my own and in my own home and in my own personal space and be successful at it.

THE DEFINITION OF COMFORT

A definition of comfort I found on the web said that 'Comfort is a sense of physical or psychological **ease**, often characterized as a lack of **hardship**'.

Persons who are lacking in comfort are uncomfortable experiencing discomfort.

A degree of psychological comfort can be achieved by recreating experiences that are associated with pleasant **memories**, such as engaging in familiar activities *of comfort.*

PIZZA BURGERS AND FRIES
YES - POSSIBLE AND HOW TO

ॐ

I just had to include this very important chapter to share because on my own personal go-to comfort food list included pizza, burgers and fries not unlike a lot of you out there. I put them all on my list so I could come up with a way to belly up these all too familiar go-to items (my bad food cognitive repeated go-to's) and here is some examples of what I did.

PIZZA

છ

Before in earlier years pizza was a huge downfall for my scale and a roadblock because I was not willing to part with my pizza. I could order and eat pizza every night for the next twenty years and still just love it. There is something about pizza that just called my name. I scoured the internet for ways to belly up pizza.

I wanted to lower the carbs, the calories, fats and or sugars but not give on the taste, texture, look or feel of regular pizza.

At first, I tried portabella mushroom cap pizzas. I must admit they were pretty good and yes, they certainly got the scale to go down. They were still smaller though and did not give me that visual in my brain of eating a regular pizza however they tasted fantastic and did get rid of the pizza craving for sure hence equalling comfort because my scale said so. So that is one of my pizza comfort food options now, however I found more pizza options and any more I found that made the scale smile got added on my go-to list so that I had multiple pizza options to choose from.

On my list also is a flax wheat crust pizza recipe so that helped me get more fiber etc. in but that version did not really cut the scale numbers that much for me personally but it was a healthier choice. Then I ran into some super belly finds, a great one being cauliflower crust pizza I found. I could eat a whole regular size pizza made out of this and the scale would smile back at me.

I used lower fat free cheese and a vegetarian version of pepperoni later on to belly it up even more and 'a-mazing'. I also ran into zucchini crust recipes and some PURE MEAT CRUST techniques and more alternatives but you get the idea I am trying to convey!

To this day I still eat pizza and if I want lots of it then I will turn to my recipes that smile on the scale at me. The comfort is definitely present, I can walk away feeling full, satiated and it tastes just as darn good as the delivered pizza and I am not missing out on anything whatsoever. Yay for cauliflower crust pizza, and chicken crust pizza, it tastes delicious and is just wonderful for so many reasons.

BURGERS

Burgers were next on my go-to list. You can load up the nutritional value menus of pretty much any type of burger from any restaurant or fast food place and see how much calories sugar carbs and fat you are consuming. I found my best number one option when I started my system was to belly up my own burgers at home until I found better outside restaurant or drive thru options. So, my next task was bellying up my own beloved burgers. I began by pulling apart my list of ingredients of what my favourite type of burger consisted of. The main burger go-to for me is usually a cheeseburger or mozzarella burger. I itemized down what was in my usual burger.

a)   Bread or bun

b)   Meat

c)   Cheese

d)   Condiments i.e.: Ketchup and Mustard

e)   Tomato Lettuce Onions

f)   Pickles

g)   Mayonnaise

At first, I could not find much for low carb, low sugar, low calorie, low fat buns on the store shelves so I opted out for low calorie bread instead. I found a brand that offers 45 calories per slice of bread so that worked as initial start but now I rarely use bread and will sometimes just use large romaine lettuce leaves to wrap my burger in – yummy. I can also use low carb almond flour bread or no bread at all and put on a plate with condiments and my pickles tomato and sometimes I like enchilada sauce on top, om-nom nom!

TIP !

After many soggy bread burgers, I finally got smart and realized the condiments do not totally soak my bread if I toast it first. I happen to like a lot of condiments so hooray for toasting and now things are working like they are supposed to. My bread does not fall apart and my burger does not fall out anymore.

Next for the patty, I purchased extra lean ground beef, mixed that with some large flake oatmeal, egg whites, some skim milk, onion powder and garlic powder and baked the patties in my oven. I make a whole batch of them and freeze like 20 burger patties at a time so I can just pull out a burger whenever the craving hits for a burger or to my hearts delight.

The cheese was pretty easy to overcome because I switched to fat free in the beginning but fat -free cheese slices do not melt so I eventually opted out for shredded block cheese instead of cheese slices. You would be amazed at how sprinkling the cheese on accomplishes the same thing as a slice of cheese taste wise but you can get the lower calories because when you sprinkle it on you will not need as much as a full slice of cheese and you are not opting out on the taste at all.

Tomatoes, onions and lettuce were nothing to belly up however I did start doubling up on these to add extra bulk to my burger and get more stuffed. So, this is a great example of where I will 'bulk it up'.

Pickles believe or not can contain a lot of salt so I went on a pickle hunt and began comparing what was available on the shelves. I located a low-salt low-calorie low carb brand of sliced pickles. Mission pickle accomplished.

Ketchup: Compare your ketchups because you can get sugar free, low sodium ketchups now and that is what I chose. They taste delicious and are lower calorie and I am not missing on any taste whatsoever.

Mustard: For mustard be careful, some are like nothing for calories and some have things added that skyrockets the calories, pick a good one for yourself that makes your scale smile at you – READ THE LABELS!

Mayonnaise was a harder hunt. I finally found a super low calorie, low sugar, low carb mayonnaise with a red lid that I personally like. It tastes yummy and works for bellying up anything with mayonnaise in it that I want (like when making devilled eggs).

So, there it is, deluxe fat juicy filling burgers that topple over if I do not physically hold them together that just stuff the crap out of me. Mission burger accomplished and the scale told me this is certainly a comfort food for me and it works very positively I can say.

TIP !

If you want bacon on your burger but not to eat too much bacon, then switch to bacon bits or you can try pork rinds crunched and sprinkled on as it becomes less calories than using full bacon strips I found if I sprinkle lightly, or alternatively I will use turkey bacon strips or turkey bacon bits when the calling hits as well.

FRIES

છ

French fries were on my go-to list as well. I initially tried chopping and baking them on a flat pan in my oven but I didn't really enjoy the taste that much or texture. They just did not seem like the fast food fries I had on my go-to list.

Then one day I learned about a machine that was a low fat multi cooker with a paddle in it that I could do fries in with just one tablespoon of oil. I watched YouTube videos and did not know anyone that had one and they were on the higher end of the price budget in the stores to get a unit so I purchased one off of a general local buy and sell board almost brand new in the box.

The lady I bought it from had used it once apparently and I paid half what I would have in the store and took it home and next I bought one of those as seen on TV potato chopping units that made perfect shaped restaurant style looking fries and loaded that up in my machine.

I added 1 tablespoon of healthy saturated fat or healthy oil to my large batch of fries and let them cook. I added some sea salt and wow, they came out golden brown and looked and tasted just so fantastic like old fashioned home made fries. I added vinegar and low sodium ketchup on them and this is now definitely an item that I can enjoy better going forward. Comfort fries and mission fries accomplished (as well variations can be done on fries of all kinds, zucchini fries and a whole whack of good nutritious foods).

I can tell you from personal experience that if my paddle machine ever breaks down, knowing what I know now, that I would definitely spend the money and go get another one from the store. I feel any machine similar like that is totally worth it to my personal comfort and peace of mind and recall me earlier in the book speaking about stocking your kitchen up with tools that make your life easier.

BULK IT UP

No matter what you choose to eat having sufficient protein is first and foremost to stay satiated. After that I can bulk it right up, the healthy way. I always without exception will try and bulk it up with healthy lower calorie, lower sugar, lower fat, lower carb and or lower salt items as much as possible. I will pile it up or pile it on; but recall portion control to.

A great aid for this is I made myself a bulk it up go-to list and put it on my fridge. Anything I chose to eat that day got a bulking up and if I was not sure what to put I would search over my list for what sounded good to me. So, if I made an egg white omelet I would add my shredded cheese but also make it loaded with my bulking personal choices. My scale quickly told me this was the right thing to do, the numbers were smiling.

For example, you could create your own bulk it up list based on your personal preferences like I did with all your favorites in it. I listed the item name, then the amount of calories approximately per item and any extra notes beside that I felt would be important to me about that item. The key for your personal bulk it up list is to pick items that you really do like the taste of but are super low in calories but packed in nutrition.

This is my own personal list I started out with and put in the book so you can get the basic idea, however eventually it is good to reorder the list for the most nutrition packed items first.

Taping the list to the fridge or cupboard door where you prepare your meals is very helpful. It catches your eye and then you look at your plate then think hmmm what else should be added that I like to bulk this up.

My personal bulk it up list looked like this however it is not yet sorted in my favorites order here (my favorites would go at the top of the list and then least at the bottom) but you get the idea as this is just an example.

Arugula: Calories: 4 per cup

Asparagus Calories: 27 per cup

Berries Calories: 32 per 1/2 cup approx. (Blueberries, raspberries, strawberries or whatever berry liked best)

Broccoli Calories: 31 per cup

Broth Calories: 10 per cup (Clear beef, chicken, miso, seafood, or vegetable broth is a secret weapon) especially if you toss in leafy greens and lean meat. Broth is the ultimate "high volume food,"

Brussel sprouts Calories: 38 per cup

Cabbage Calories: 22 per cup

Lettuce Calories: 5 per cup

Beets Calories: 37 per 1/2 cup

Cauliflower calories: 25 per cup

Black Coffee Calories: zero

Grapefruit Calories: 39 per half fruit

Remember the Grapefruit Diet? I read that studies reveal that, on average, women who consumed any amount of grapefruit or grapefruit juice weighed nearly 10 pounds less and had a 6 percent lower body mass index (BMI) than non-grapefruit-eating women and that it helps metabolism.

Mushrooms Calories: 15 per cup

Tomatoes Calories: 22 per medium tomato

Turnips Calories: 36 per cup

(The potatoes skinnier cousin, turnips are a great source of fiber and vitamin C and have a lower glycemic load. They are tasty when diced and tossed into soups or stews or baked with fat free sour cream on them.)

Watercress Calories: 4 per cup (A cleansing cruciferous vegetable with the fresh crunch of salad)

Zucchini Calories: 20 per cup

(This miracle squash is the ultimate high volume food, meaning you can fill up on very few calories.)

Spinach Calories: 7 per cup

Lemons and limes Calories: 20 per fruit (without peel)

Kale Calories: 5 per cup

Garlic Calories: 4 per clove

Peppers Calories: 30 per half cup

Onions Calories: 32 per half cup

Pumpkin Calories: 30 per cup

Radishes Calories: 19 per cup

Black Tea Calories: 0

Fennel Calories: 27 per cup

Celery Calories: 16 per cup (Crunchy, packed with fiber and an incredibly high-volume food meaning you can eat a lot for a few calories; celery is a chef's secret weapon.)

Carrots Calories: 22 per 1/2 cup

CHAPTER 4

$$\text{ED}$$

THE FULL BELLY SYSTEM
QUICK STEP START LIST

N ow that you have read the important keys and you have an idea how this is going to work and see just what I did on my system to get success here is just a quick recap in simplified steps to refresh.

PREPARATION SUGGESTIONS:

- ✓ Selfie photos taken if you want to.
- ✓ Pair of shorts or sweats with drawstring tied as described earlier in the book. Or use a tape measure if you prefer.
- ✓ Digital Scale.

Think about this statement...

"IF YOU ARE EXERCISING JUST TO EAT THEN YOU NEED TO RE-EVALUATE YOUR PRIORITIES"

Now think about this too...

"A HOLIDAY IS NOT A COUPLE OF WEEKS, NOR A COUPLE OF DAYS. AS THE WORD SAYS IT IS A 'HOLI – DAY'. JUST ONE SINGLE DAY. NOT WEEKS, NOT DAYS, SO HENCE YOU CAN EVEN DEFINE THAT DOWN FURTHER TO REALIZE IT IS USUALLY JUST A DINNER FOR A FEW HOURS."

STARTING THE WORKBOOK PAGES

ෂ්

STEP 1

Suggested: Eating normally for the first 1-3 days. Eating enough to not be sick but to be able to know the stuffed thought hit the brain. That is the full belly meter signal to the brain – the braintrain. Starting on a weekend is just fine because there is no real work being done here yet.

STEP 2

Suggested: Record morning weight around the same time each morning for the next 30-60-90 days or longer if you wish – recall it is your choice how long you feel you need to record for.

STEP 3

Suggested: For each day; record everything you eat. You may wish to include calorie counting or any other counting you wish but mark it down what you ate or drank for sure so you can belly this stuff up later.

STEP 4

Suggested: Record your evening or bedtime weight around the same time each evening for the next 30-60 days or longer if you wish. Remember this number will always be higher than your morning weight.

STEP 5

Suggested: Create your regular routine go-to comfort food list which is sure to be full of calories, fats, sugars and salts in the start. Be sure to write down all your favourites in order of importance to you. This is one of the 'super keys' to succeeding on the full belly meter system. Include all regular foods or drinks you love and eat most often. List them in or of highest priority to you with lowest priority being last on the list.

STEP 6

Suggested: Create your bulk it up list and put that on your fridge door for reference whenever you need, use it as a reminder as well.

STEP 7

Suggested: Continue your morning and evening weighing and recording what you ate. Start bellying up your personal go-to or favourite foods list. You need to make your list comfortable for each item on that list.

To make it comfortable means to belly it up, calorie it down, use substitutes, lower carb, healthy fats, nutritional fats, salt or sugar it down as much as possible or whatever you can do to improve on it and try to do this without losing your look, feel, texture or taste as much as possible so your body doesn't even realize you are missing the fat normally added to your body while you eat healthy and satisfied to yourself each day. Remember that bulking it up can be very helpful and rewarding to bellying up a recipe. Ask for help from your doctor or registered dietician if you are not sure what is best for you or if you would like a detailed plan just for you.

STEP 8

Suggested: In the workbook pages write down the time you ate, what you ate next, any calorie amount or other counting method or system you are currently using, and then record your belly meter level after you ate as:

1) Hungry – meaning you are still wanting food, still feeling hungry.

2) Full – meaning you are feeling full.

3) Just stuffed – meaning you cannot take in another bite and your stomach is telling your brain I am stuffed – stop eating. (Never abuse this step).

STEP 9

Suggested: Repeat until you get some positive results like I did. Once you start seeing some positives look at what you did and stick with it or improve even more on it. If my numbers stayed the same on the scale, I had to review my foods I consumed and see what I could improve on.

STEP 10

Suggested: Remember to get your draw string shorts or sweats in order and to snap your selfie shots. Organize your kitchen, cupboards, freezer and fridge to set yourself up for success. Organize all lists like your favourite foods list and your bulk it up list.

TIP !

Watch out as you go for hidden calories you are not aware of. For example, I learned a big surprise one day which was my favourite coffee place – I was using 2 creams in each coffee that were totalling 180 calories per day and had no idea how fattening that cream really was. I switched to 2 milks instead and my coffee dropped to 40 calories per coffee instead of 180. I read it takes a deficit of approximately 3500 calories to lose 1 pound so that was a no brainer in my mind to switch to milk instead of cream in the beginning.

Also remember if you are going out to eat you can google restaurant menus for the menu list and nutritional value of the menu items before you get there so you can plan ahead what you want. You should pick about 2 to 3 dishes of your best choices in case they are out of one dish when you arrive, at least you will have your back up plan in place. If required, bring your own dressing with you as a lot of restaurant dressings may not be what you are seeking to get to your goal. Now you are ready to begin your new journey.

Dear Weighted,

I sincerely hope you benefit from this system as I have. It is my wish for you that I am able to put a smile on your scale and a smile on your face now and for many years to come. You are in this for the long haul this time, just like me and this is so well worth it! Results may vary per individual nutritional choices and I am sure you will know what the better choices for you are going to be moving forward today. This system forces you to be very accountable to yourself yet is not a difficult or expensive system to learn.

Should you want to drop the author a message on how you are doing, a comment or if you have a question on something then please do so by visiting the website at **www.fullbellymeter.com** .

Most Sincerely,

Katherine

THE FULL BELLY METER

WORKBOOK SECTION

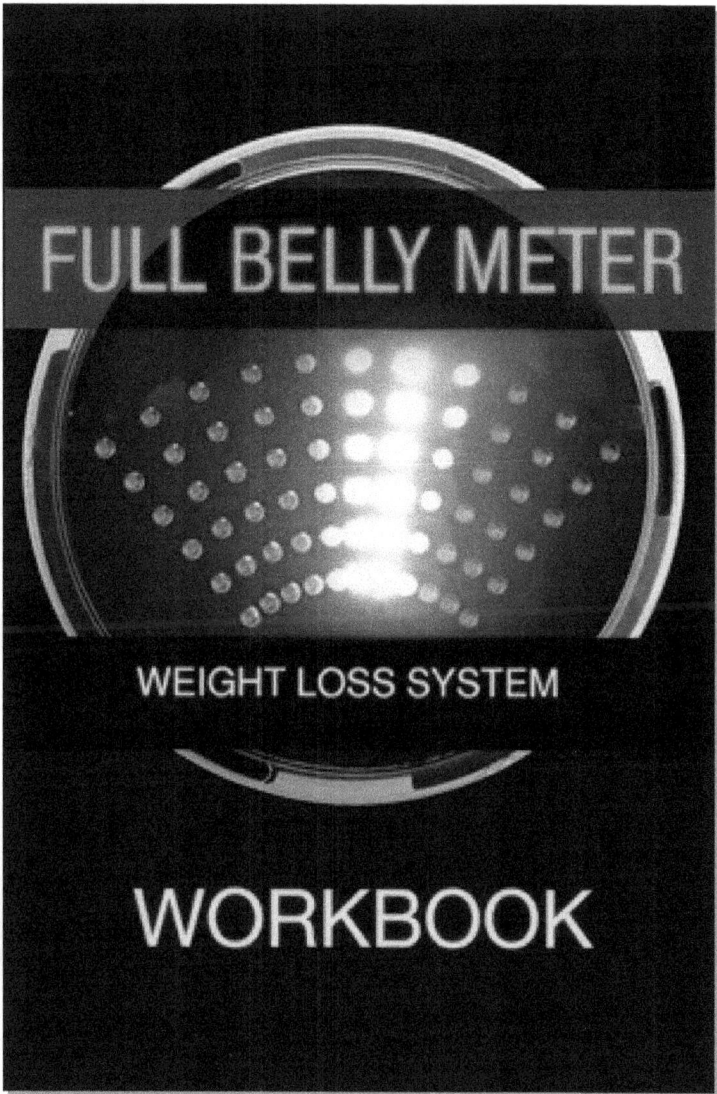

MORNING WEIGHT

DATE - DAILY FOOD JOURNAL

FULL BELLY METER WORKBOOK

RECORD THE TIME, ITEM, ANY COUNTS YOU ARE DOING, AND YOUR METER LEVEL YOU FELT AFTER EATING. REMEMBER TO HAVE AN ADEQUATE AMOUNT OF PROTEIN TO SUSTAIN SATIETY (FEELING FULLER LONGER), CHOOSE THE GOOD FATS, CHOOSE THE GOOD CARBS AS YOU GO.

Time	Food & Drink Intake	Cal/Carbs/Sugar/Other	Meter Level
			›HUNGRY
			›FULL
			›JUST STUFFED

NIGHT WEIGHT

_____
MORNING WEIGHT

_____
DATE - DAILY FOOD JOURNAL

FULL BELLY METER WORKBOOK

RECORD THE TIME, ITEM, ANY COUNTS YOU ARE DOING, AND YOUR
METER LEVEL YOU FELT AFTER EATING. REMEMBER TO HAVE AN
ADEQUATE AMOUNT OF PROTEIN TO SUSTAIN SATIETY (FEELING
FULLER LONGER), CHOOSE THE GOOD FATS, CHOOSE THE GOOD
CARBS AS YOU GO.

Time	Food & Drink Intake	Cal/Carbs/Sugar/Other	Meter Level
			>HUNGRY
			>FULL
			>JUST STUFFED

_____
NIGHT WEIGHT

_____
MORNING WEIGHT

_____
DATE - DAILY FOOD JOURNAL

FULL BELLY METER WORKBOOK

RECORD THE TIME, ITEM, ANY COUNTS YOU ARE DOING, AND YOUR
METER LEVEL YOU FELT AFTER EATING. REMEMBER TO HAVE AN
ADEQUATE AMOUNT OF PROTEIN TO SUSTAIN SATIETY (FEELING
FULLER LONGER), CHOOSE THE GOOD FATS, CHOOSE THE GOOD
CARBS AS YOU GO.

Time	Food & Drink Intake	Cal/Carbs/Sugar/Other	Meter Level
			›HUNGRY
			›FULL
			›JUST STUFFED

_____
NIGHT WEIGHT

_____
MORNING WEIGHT

_____
DATE - DAILY FOOD JOURNAL

FULL BELLY METER WORKBOOK

RECORD THE TIME, ITEM, ANY COUNTS YOU ARE DOING, AND YOUR
METER LEVEL YOU FELT AFTER EATING. REMEMBER TO HAVE AN
ADEQUATE AMOUNT OF PROTEIN TO SUSTAIN SATIETY (FEELING
FULLER LONGER), CHOOSE THE GOOD FATS, CHOOSE THE GOOD
CARBS AS YOU GO.

Time	Food & Drink Intake	Cal/Carbs/Sugar/Other	Meter Level
			>HUNGRY
			>FULL
			>JUST STUFFED

_____
NIGHT WEIGHT

MORNING WEIGHT

DATE - DAILY FOOD JOURNAL

FULL BELLY METER WORKBOOK

RECORD THE TIME, ITEM, ANY COUNTS YOU ARE DOING, AND YOUR
METER LEVEL YOU FELT AFTER EATING. REMEMBER TO HAVE AN
ADEQUATE AMOUNT OF PROTEIN TO SUSTAIN SATIETY (FEELING
FULLER LONGER), CHOOSE THE GOOD FATS, CHOOSE THE GOOD
CARBS AS YOU GO.

Time	Food & Drink Intake	Cal/Carbs/Sugar/Other	Meter Level
			›HUNGRY
			›FULL
			›JUST STUFFED

NIGHT WEIGHT

MORNING WEIGHT

DATE - DAILY FOOD JOURNAL

FULL BELLY METER WORKBOOK

RECORD THE TIME, ITEM, ANY COUNTS YOU ARE DOING, AND YOUR METER LEVEL YOU FELT AFTER EATING. REMEMBER TO HAVE AN ADEQUATE AMOUNT OF PROTEIN TO SUSTAIN SATIETY (FEELING FULLER LONGER), CHOOSE THE GOOD FATS, CHOOSE THE GOOD CARBS AS YOU GO.

Time	Food & Drink Intake	Cal/Carbs/Sugar/Other	Meter Level
			>HUNGRY
			>FULL
			>JUST STUFFED

NIGHT WEIGHT

_____   _____
MORNING WEIGHT   DATE - DAILY FOOD JOURNAL

FULL BELLY METER WORKBOOK

RECORD THE TIME, ITEM, ANY COUNTS YOU ARE DOING, AND YOUR
METER LEVEL YOU FELT AFTER EATING. REMEMBER TO HAVE AN
ADEQUATE AMOUNT OF PROTEIN TO SUSTAIN SATIETY (FEELING
FULLER LONGER), CHOOSE THE GOOD FATS, CHOOSE THE GOOD
CARBS AS YOU GO.

Time	Food & Drink Intake	Cal/Carbs/Sugar/Other	Meter Level
			›HUNGRY
			›FULL
			›JUST STUFFED

_____
NIGHT WEIGHT

MORNING WEIGHT

DATE - DAILY FOOD JOURNAL

FULL BELLY METER WORKBOOK

RECORD THE TIME, ITEM, ANY COUNTS YOU ARE DOING, AND YOUR
METER LEVEL YOU FELT AFTER EATING. REMEMBER TO HAVE AN
ADEQUATE AMOUNT OF PROTEIN TO SUSTAIN SATIETY (FEELING
FULLER LONGER), CHOOSE THE GOOD FATS, CHOOSE THE GOOD
CARBS AS YOU GO.

Time	Food & Drink Intake	Cal/Carbs/Sugar/Other	Meter Level
			>HUNGRY
			>FULL
			>JUST STUFFED

NIGHT WEIGHT

MORNING WEIGHT

DATE - DAILY FOOD JOURNAL

FULL BELLY METER WORKBOOK

RECORD THE TIME, ITEM, ANY COUNTS YOU ARE DOING, AND YOUR
METER LEVEL YOU FELT AFTER EATING. REMEMBER TO HAVE AN
ADEQUATE AMOUNT OF PROTEIN TO SUSTAIN SATIETY (FEELING
FULLER LONGER), CHOOSE THE GOOD FATS, CHOOSE THE GOOD
CARBS AS YOU GO.

Time	Food & Drink Intake	Cal/Carbs/Sugar/Other	Meter Level
			>HUNGRY
			>FULL
			>JUST STUFFED

NIGHT WEIGHT

MORNING WEIGHT

DATE - DAILY FOOD JOURNAL

FULL BELLY METER WORKBOOK

RECORD THE TIME, ITEM, ANY COUNTS YOU ARE DOING, AND YOUR METER LEVEL YOU FELT AFTER EATING. REMEMBER TO HAVE AN ADEQUATE AMOUNT OF PROTEIN TO SUSTAIN SATIETY (FEELING FULLER LONGER), CHOOSE THE GOOD FATS, CHOOSE THE GOOD CARBS AS YOU GO.

Time	Food & Drink Intake	Cal/Carbs/Sugar/Other	Meter Level
			>HUNGRY >FULL >JUST STUFFED

NIGHT WEIGHT

MORNING WEIGHT

DATE - DAILY FOOD JOURNAL

FULL BELLY METER WORKBOOK

RECORD THE TIME, ITEM, ANY COUNTS YOU ARE DOING, AND YOUR
METER LEVEL YOU FELT AFTER EATING. REMEMBER TO HAVE AN
ADEQUATE AMOUNT OF PROTEIN TO SUSTAIN SATIETY (FEELING
FULLER LONGER), CHOOSE THE GOOD FATS, CHOOSE THE GOOD
CARBS AS YOU GO.

Time	Food & Drink Intake	Cal/Carbs/Sugar/Other	Meter Level
			>HUNGRY
			>FULL
			>JUST STUFFED

NIGHT WEIGHT

MORNING WEIGHT   DATE - DAILY FOOD JOURNAL

FULL BELLY METER WORKBOOK

RECORD THE TIME, ITEM, ANY COUNTS YOU ARE DOING, AND YOUR
METER LEVEL YOU FELT AFTER EATING. REMEMBER TO HAVE AN
ADEQUATE AMOUNT OF PROTEIN TO SUSTAIN SATIETY (FEELING
FULLER LONGER), CHOOSE THE GOOD FATS, CHOOSE THE GOOD
CARBS AS YOU GO.

Time	Food & Drink Intake	Cal/Carbs/Sugar/Other	Meter Level
			>HUNGRY
			>FULL
			>JUST STUFFED

NIGHT WEIGHT

MORNING WEIGHT

DATE - DAILY FOOD JOURNAL

FULL BELLY METER WORKBOOK

RECORD THE TIME, ITEM, ANY COUNTS YOU ARE DOING, AND YOUR METER LEVEL YOU FELT AFTER EATING. REMEMBER TO HAVE AN ADEQUATE AMOUNT OF PROTEIN TO SUSTAIN SATIETY (FEELING FULLER LONGER), CHOOSE THE GOOD FATS, CHOOSE THE GOOD CARBS AS YOU GO.

Time	Food & Drink Intake	Cal/Carbs/Sugar/Other	Meter Level
			›HUNGRY ›FULL ›JUST STUFFED

NIGHT WEIGHT

MORNING WEIGHT

DATE - DAILY FOOD JOURNAL

FULL BELLY METER WORKBOOK

RECORD THE TIME, ITEM, ANY COUNTS YOU ARE DOING, AND YOUR
METER LEVEL YOU FELT AFTER EATING. REMEMBER TO HAVE AN
ADEQUATE AMOUNT OF PROTEIN TO SUSTAIN SATIETY (FEELING
FULLER LONGER), CHOOSE THE GOOD FATS, CHOOSE THE GOOD
CARBS AS YOU GO.

Time	Food & Drink Intake	Cal/Carbs/Sugar/Other	Meter Level
			>HUNGRY
			>FULL
			>JUST STUFFED

NIGHT WEIGHT

MORNING WEIGHT

DATE - DAILY FOOD JOURNAL

FULL BELLY METER WORKBOOK

RECORD THE TIME, ITEM, ANY COUNTS YOU ARE DOING, AND YOUR METER LEVEL YOU FELT AFTER EATING. REMEMBER TO HAVE AN ADEQUATE AMOUNT OF PROTEIN TO SUSTAIN SATIETY (FEELING FULLER LONGER), CHOOSE THE GOOD FATS, CHOOSE THE GOOD CARBS AS YOU GO.

Time	Food & Drink Intake	Cal/Carbs/Sugar/Other	Meter Level
			>HUNGRY
			>FULL
			>JUST STUFFED

NIGHT WEIGHT

MORNING WEIGHT

DATE - DAILY FOOD JOURNAL

FULL BELLY METER WORKBOOK

RECORD THE TIME, ITEM, ANY COUNTS YOU ARE DOING, AND YOUR METER LEVEL YOU FELT AFTER EATING. REMEMBER TO HAVE AN ADEQUATE AMOUNT OF PROTEIN TO SUSTAIN SATIETY (FEELING FULLER LONGER), CHOOSE THE GOOD FATS, CHOOSE THE GOOD CARBS AS YOU GO.

Time	Food & Drink Intake	Cal/Carbs/Sugar/Other	Meter Level
			>HUNGRY
			>FULL
			>JUST STUFFED

NIGHT WEIGHT

_____   _____
MORNING WEIGHT   DATE - DAILY FOOD JOURNAL

FULL BELLY METER WORKBOOK

RECORD THE TIME, ITEM, ANY COUNTS YOU ARE DOING, AND YOUR
METER LEVEL YOU FELT AFTER EATING. REMEMBER TO HAVE AN
ADEQUATE AMOUNT OF PROTEIN TO SUSTAIN SATIETY (FEELING
FULLER LONGER), CHOOSE THE GOOD FATS, CHOOSE THE GOOD
CARBS AS YOU GO.

Time	Food & Drink Intake	Cal/Carbs/Sugar/Other	Meter Level
			›HUNGRY
			›FULL
			›JUST STUFFED

_____
NIGHT WEIGHT

MORNING WEIGHT

DATE - DAILY FOOD JOURNAL

FULL BELLY METER WORKBOOK

RECORD THE TIME, ITEM, ANY COUNTS YOU ARE DOING, AND YOUR METER LEVEL YOU FELT AFTER EATING. REMEMBER TO HAVE AN ADEQUATE AMOUNT OF PROTEIN TO SUSTAIN SATIETY (FEELING FULLER LONGER), CHOOSE THE GOOD FATS, CHOOSE THE GOOD CARBS AS YOU GO.

Time	Food & Drink Intake	Cal/Carbs/Sugar/Other	Meter Level
			>HUNGRY
			>FULL
			>JUST STUFFED

NIGHT WEIGHT

MORNING WEIGHT

DATE - DAILY FOOD JOURNAL

FULL BELLY METER WORKBOOK

RECORD THE TIME, ITEM, ANY COUNTS YOU ARE DOING, AND YOUR
METER LEVEL YOU FELT AFTER EATING. REMEMBER TO HAVE AN
ADEQUATE AMOUNT OF PROTEIN TO SUSTAIN SATIETY (FEELING
FULLER LONGER), CHOOSE THE GOOD FATS, CHOOSE THE GOOD
CARBS AS YOU GO.

Time	Food & Drink Intake	Cal/Carbs/Sugar/Other	Meter Level
			›HUNGRY
			›FULL
			›JUST STUFFED

NIGHT WEIGHT

MORNING WEIGHT

DATE - DAILY FOOD JOURNAL

FULL BELLY METER WORKBOOK

RECORD THE TIME, ITEM, ANY COUNTS YOU ARE DOING, AND YOUR
METER LEVEL YOU FELT AFTER EATING. REMEMBER TO HAVE AN
ADEQUATE AMOUNT OF PROTEIN TO SUSTAIN SATIETY (FEELING
FULLER LONGER), CHOOSE THE GOOD FATS, CHOOSE THE GOOD
CARBS AS YOU GO.

Time	Food & Drink Intake	Cal/Carbs/Sugar/Other	Meter Level
			>HUNGRY
			>FULL
			>JUST STUFFED

NIGHT WEIGHT

MORNING WEIGHT

DATE - DAILY FOOD JOURNAL

FULL BELLY METER WORKBOOK

RECORD THE TIME, ITEM, ANY COUNTS YOU ARE DOING, AND YOUR
METER LEVEL YOU FELT AFTER EATING. REMEMBER TO HAVE AN
ADEQUATE AMOUNT OF PROTEIN TO SUSTAIN SATIETY (FEELING
FULLER LONGER), CHOOSE THE GOOD FATS, CHOOSE THE GOOD
CARBS AS YOU GO.

Time	Food & Drink Intake	Cal/Carbs/Sugar/Other	Meter Level
			>HUNGRY
			>FULL
			>JUST STUFFED

NIGHT WEIGHT

MORNING WEIGHT

DATE - DAILY FOOD JOURNAL

FULL BELLY METER WORKBOOK

RECORD THE TIME, ITEM, ANY COUNTS YOU ARE DOING, AND YOUR METER LEVEL YOU FELT AFTER EATING. REMEMBER TO HAVE AN ADEQUATE AMOUNT OF PROTEIN TO SUSTAIN SATIETY (FEELING FULLER LONGER), CHOOSE THE GOOD FATS, CHOOSE THE GOOD CARBS AS YOU GO.

Time	Food & Drink Intake	Cal/Carbs/Sugar/Other	Meter Level
			>HUNGRY
			>FULL
			>JUST STUFFED

NIGHT WEIGHT

_____
MORNING WEIGHT

_____
DATE - DAILY FOOD JOURNAL

FULL BELLY METER WORKBOOK

RECORD THE TIME, ITEM, ANY COUNTS YOU ARE DOING, AND YOUR
METER LEVEL YOU FELT AFTER EATING. REMEMBER TO HAVE AN
ADEQUATE AMOUNT OF PROTEIN TO SUSTAIN SATIETY (FEELING
FULLER LONGER), CHOOSE THE GOOD FATS, CHOOSE THE GOOD
CARBS AS YOU GO.

Time	Food & Drink Intake	Cal/Carbs/Sugar/Other	Meter Level
			>HUNGRY
			>FULL
			>JUST STUFFED

_____
NIGHT WEIGHT

MORNING WEIGHT

DATE - DAILY FOOD JOURNAL

FULL BELLY METER WORKBOOK

RECORD THE TIME, ITEM, ANY COUNTS YOU ARE DOING, AND YOUR METER LEVEL YOU FELT AFTER EATING. REMEMBER TO HAVE AN ADEQUATE AMOUNT OF PROTEIN TO SUSTAIN SATIETY (FEELING FULLER LONGER), CHOOSE THE GOOD FATS, CHOOSE THE GOOD CARBS AS YOU GO.

Time	Food & Drink Intake	Cal/Carbs/Sugar/Other	Meter Level
			>HUNGRY
			>FULL
			>JUST STUFFED

NIGHT WEIGHT

MORNING WEIGHT

DATE - DAILY FOOD JOURNAL

FULL BELLY METER WORKBOOK

RECORD THE TIME, ITEM, ANY COUNTS YOU ARE DOING, AND YOUR METER LEVEL YOU FELT AFTER EATING. REMEMBER TO HAVE AN ADEQUATE AMOUNT OF PROTEIN TO SUSTAIN SATIETY (FEELING FULLER LONGER), CHOOSE THE GOOD FATS, CHOOSE THE GOOD CARBS AS YOU GO.

Time	Food & Drink Intake	Cal/Carbs/Sugar/Other	Meter Level
			›HUNGRY ›FULL ›JUST STUFFED

NIGHT WEIGHT

_____   _____
MORNING WEIGHT   DATE - DAILY FOOD JOURNAL

FULL BELLY METER WORKBOOK

RECORD THE TIME, ITEM, ANY COUNTS YOU ARE DOING, AND YOUR
METER LEVEL YOU FELT AFTER EATING. REMEMBER TO HAVE AN
ADEQUATE AMOUNT OF PROTEIN TO SUSTAIN SATIETY (FEELING
FULLER LONGER), CHOOSE THE GOOD FATS, CHOOSE THE GOOD
CARBS AS YOU GO.

Time	Food & Drink Intake	Cal/Carbs/Sugar/Other	Meter Level
			>HUNGRY
			>FULL
			>JUST STUFFED

_____
NIGHT WEIGHT

MORNING WEIGHT

DATE - DAILY FOOD JOURNAL

FULL BELLY METER WORKBOOK

RECORD THE TIME, ITEM, ANY COUNTS YOU ARE DOING, AND YOUR METER LEVEL YOU FELT AFTER EATING. REMEMBER TO HAVE AN ADEQUATE AMOUNT OF PROTEIN TO SUSTAIN SATIETY (FEELING FULLER LONGER), CHOOSE THE GOOD FATS, CHOOSE THE GOOD CARBS AS YOU GO.

Time	Food & Drink Intake	Cal/Carbs/Sugar/Other	Meter Level
			>HUNGRY
			>FULL
			>JUST STUFFED

NIGHT WEIGHT

_____
MORNING WEIGHT

_____
DATE - DAILY FOOD JOURNAL

FULL BELLY METER WORKBOOK

RECORD THE TIME, ITEM, ANY COUNTS YOU ARE DOING, AND YOUR
METER LEVEL YOU FELT AFTER EATING. REMEMBER TO HAVE AN
ADEQUATE AMOUNT OF PROTEIN TO SUSTAIN SATIETY (FEELING
FULLER LONGER), CHOOSE THE GOOD FATS, CHOOSE THE GOOD
CARBS AS YOU GO.

Time	Food & Drink Intake	Cal/Carbs/Sugar/Other	Meter Level
			>HUNGRY
			>FULL
			>JUST STUFFED

_____
NIGHT WEIGHT

<u>MORNING WEIGHT</u>   <u>DATE - DAILY FOOD JOURNAL</u>

FULL BELLY METER WORKBOOK

RECORD THE TIME, ITEM, ANY COUNTS YOU ARE DOING, AND YOUR
METER LEVEL YOU FELT AFTER EATING. REMEMBER TO HAVE AN
ADEQUATE AMOUNT OF PROTEIN TO SUSTAIN SATIETY (FEELING
FULLER LONGER), CHOOSE THE GOOD FATS, CHOOSE THE GOOD
CARBS AS YOU GO.

Time	Food & Drink Intake	Cal/Carbs/Sugar/Other	Meter Level
			>HUNGRY
			>FULL
			>JUST STUFFED

<u>NIGHT WEIGHT</u>

_____   _____

MORNING WEIGHT   DATE - DAILY FOOD JOURNAL

FULL BELLY METER WORKBOOK

RECORD THE TIME, ITEM, ANY COUNTS YOU ARE DOING, AND YOUR
METER LEVEL YOU FELT AFTER EATING. REMEMBER TO HAVE AN
ADEQUATE AMOUNT OF PROTEIN TO SUSTAIN SATIETY (FEELING
FULLER LONGER), CHOOSE THE GOOD FATS, CHOOSE THE GOOD
CARBS AS YOU GO.

Time	Food & Drink Intake	Cal/Carbs/Sugar/Other	Meter Level
			>HUNGRY
			>FULL
			>JUST STUFFED

_____

NIGHT WEIGHT

_____
MORNING WEIGHT

_____
DATE - DAILY FOOD JOURNAL

FULL BELLY METER WORKBOOK

RECORD THE TIME, ITEM, ANY COUNTS YOU ARE DOING, AND YOUR METER LEVEL YOU FELT AFTER EATING. REMEMBER TO HAVE AN ADEQUATE AMOUNT OF PROTEIN TO SUSTAIN SATIETY (FEELING FULLER LONGER), CHOOSE THE GOOD FATS, CHOOSE THE GOOD CARBS AS YOU GO.

Time	Food & Drink Intake	Cal/Carbs/Sugar/Other	Meter Level
			›HUNGRY
			›FULL
			›JUST STUFFED

_____
NIGHT WEIGHT

_____
MORNING WEIGHT

_____
DATE - DAILY FOOD JOURNAL

FULL BELLY METER WORKBOOK

RECORD THE TIME, ITEM, ANY COUNTS YOU ARE DOING, AND YOUR METER LEVEL YOU FELT AFTER EATING. REMEMBER TO HAVE AN ADEQUATE AMOUNT OF PROTEIN TO SUSTAIN SATIETY (FEELING FULLER LONGER), CHOOSE THE GOOD FATS, CHOOSE THE GOOD CARBS AS YOU GO.

Time	Food & Drink Intake	Cal/Carbs/Sugar/Other	Meter Level
			>HUNGRY
			>FULL
			>JUST STUFFED

_____
NIGHT WEIGHT

MORNING WEIGHT

DATE - DAILY FOOD JOURNAL

FULL BELLY METER WORKBOOK

RECORD THE TIME, ITEM, ANY COUNTS YOU ARE DOING, AND YOUR METER LEVEL YOU FELT AFTER EATING. REMEMBER TO HAVE AN ADEQUATE AMOUNT OF PROTEIN TO SUSTAIN SATIETY (FEELING FULLER LONGER), CHOOSE THE GOOD FATS, CHOOSE THE GOOD CARBS AS YOU GO.

Time	Food & Drink Intake	Cal/Carbs/Sugar/Other	Meter Level
			>HUNGRY
			>FULL
			>JUST STUFFED

NIGHT WEIGHT

MORNING WEIGHT

DATE - DAILY FOOD JOURNAL

FULL BELLY METER WORKBOOK

RECORD THE TIME, ITEM, ANY COUNTS YOU ARE DOING, AND YOUR METER LEVEL YOU FELT AFTER EATING. REMEMBER TO HAVE AN ADEQUATE AMOUNT OF PROTEIN TO SUSTAIN SATIETY (FEELING FULLER LONGER), CHOOSE THE GOOD FATS, CHOOSE THE GOOD CARBS AS YOU GO.

Time	Food & Drink Intake	Cal/Carbs/Sugar/Other	Meter Level
			>HUNGRY
			>FULL
			>JUST STUFFED

NIGHT WEIGHT

MORNING WEIGHT

DATE - DAILY FOOD JOURNAL

FULL BELLY METER WORKBOOK

RECORD THE TIME, ITEM, ANY COUNTS YOU ARE DOING, AND YOUR
METER LEVEL YOU FELT AFTER EATING. REMEMBER TO HAVE AN
ADEQUATE AMOUNT OF PROTEIN TO SUSTAIN SATIETY (FEELING
FULLER LONGER), CHOOSE THE GOOD FATS, CHOOSE THE GOOD
CARBS AS YOU GO.

Time	Food & Drink Intake	Cal/Carbs/Sugar/Other	Meter Level
			›HUNGRY
			›FULL
			›JUST STUFFED

NIGHT WEIGHT

MORNING WEIGHT

DATE - DAILY FOOD JOURNAL

FULL BELLY METER WORKBOOK

RECORD THE TIME, ITEM, ANY COUNTS YOU ARE DOING, AND YOUR METER LEVEL YOU FELT AFTER EATING. REMEMBER TO HAVE AN ADEQUATE AMOUNT OF PROTEIN TO SUSTAIN SATIETY (FEELING FULLER LONGER), CHOOSE THE GOOD FATS, CHOOSE THE GOOD CARBS AS YOU GO.

Time	Food & Drink Intake	Cal/Carbs/Sugar/Other	Meter Level
			>HUNGRY
			>FULL
			>JUST STUFFED

NIGHT WEIGHT

MORNING WEIGHT

DATE - DAILY FOOD JOURNAL

FULL BELLY METER WORKBOOK

RECORD THE TIME, ITEM, ANY COUNTS YOU ARE DOING, AND YOUR
METER LEVEL YOU FELT AFTER EATING. REMEMBER TO HAVE AN
ADEQUATE AMOUNT OF PROTEIN TO SUSTAIN SATIETY (FEELING
FULLER LONGER), CHOOSE THE GOOD FATS, CHOOSE THE GOOD
CARBS AS YOU GO.

Time	Food & Drink Intake	Cal/Carbs/Sugar/Other	Meter Level
			›HUNGRY
			›FULL
			›JUST STUFFED

NIGHT WEIGHT

MORNING WEIGHT

DATE - DAILY FOOD JOURNAL

FULL BELLY METER WORKBOOK

RECORD THE TIME, ITEM, ANY COUNTS YOU ARE DOING, AND YOUR
METER LEVEL YOU FELT AFTER EATING. REMEMBER TO HAVE AN
ADEQUATE AMOUNT OF PROTEIN TO SUSTAIN SATIETY (FEELING
FULLER LONGER), CHOOSE THE GOOD FATS, CHOOSE THE GOOD
CARBS AS YOU GO.

Time	Food & Drink Intake	Cal/Carbs/Sugar/Other	Meter Level
			>HUNGRY
			>FULL
			>JUST STUFFED

NIGHT WEIGHT

_____   _____
MORNING WEIGHT   DATE - DAILY FOOD JOURNAL

FULL BELLY METER WORKBOOK

RECORD THE TIME, ITEM, ANY COUNTS YOU ARE DOING, AND YOUR
METER LEVEL YOU FELT AFTER EATING. REMEMBER TO HAVE AN
ADEQUATE AMOUNT OF PROTEIN TO SUSTAIN SATIETY (FEELING
FULLER LONGER), CHOOSE THE GOOD FATS, CHOOSE THE GOOD
CARBS AS YOU GO.

Time	Food & Drink Intake	Cal/Carbs/Sugar/Other	Meter Level
			>HUNGRY
			>FULL
			>JUST STUFFED

_____
NIGHT WEIGHT

MORNING WEIGHT

DATE - DAILY FOOD JOURNAL

FULL BELLY METER WORKBOOK

RECORD THE TIME, ITEM, ANY COUNTS YOU ARE DOING, AND YOUR METER LEVEL YOU FELT AFTER EATING. REMEMBER TO HAVE AN ADEQUATE AMOUNT OF PROTEIN TO SUSTAIN SATIETY (FEELING FULLER LONGER), CHOOSE THE GOOD FATS, CHOOSE THE GOOD CARBS AS YOU GO.

Time	Food & Drink Intake	Cal/Carbs/Sugar/Other	Meter Level
			>HUNGRY
			>FULL
			>JUST STUFFED

NIGHT WEIGHT

MORNING WEIGHT   DATE - DAILY FOOD JOURNAL

FULL BELLY METER WORKBOOK

RECORD THE TIME, ITEM, ANY COUNTS YOU ARE DOING, AND YOUR
METER LEVEL YOU FELT AFTER EATING. REMEMBER TO HAVE AN
ADEQUATE AMOUNT OF PROTEIN TO SUSTAIN SATIETY (FEELING
FULLER LONGER), CHOOSE THE GOOD FATS, CHOOSE THE GOOD
CARBS AS YOU GO.

Time	Food & Drink Intake	Cal/Carbs/Sugar/Other	Meter Level
			>HUNGRY
			>FULL
			>JUST STUFFED

NIGHT WEIGHT

_____   _____

MORNING WEIGHT   DATE - DAILY FOOD JOURNAL

FULL BELLY METER WORKBOOK

RECORD THE TIME, ITEM, ANY COUNTS YOU ARE DOING, AND YOUR
METER LEVEL YOU FELT AFTER EATING. REMEMBER TO HAVE AN
ADEQUATE AMOUNT OF PROTEIN TO SUSTAIN SATIETY (FEELING
FULLER LONGER), CHOOSE THE GOOD FATS, CHOOSE THE GOOD
CARBS AS YOU GO.

Time	Food & Drink Intake	Cal/Carbs/Sugar/Other	Meter Level
			>HUNGRY
			>FULL
			>JUST STUFFED

_____

NIGHT WEIGHT

MORNING WEIGHT

DATE - DAILY FOOD JOURNAL

FULL BELLY METER WORKBOOK

RECORD THE TIME, ITEM, ANY COUNTS YOU ARE DOING, AND YOUR METER LEVEL YOU FELT AFTER EATING. REMEMBER TO HAVE AN ADEQUATE AMOUNT OF PROTEIN TO SUSTAIN SATIETY (FEELING FULLER LONGER), CHOOSE THE GOOD FATS, CHOOSE THE GOOD CARBS AS YOU GO.

Time	Food & Drink Intake	Cal/Carbs/Sugar/Other	Meter Level
			›HUNGRY
			›FULL
			›JUST STUFFED

NIGHT WEIGHT

MORNING WEIGHT   DATE - DAILY FOOD JOURNAL

FULL BELLY METER WORKBOOK

RECORD THE TIME, ITEM, ANY COUNTS YOU ARE DOING, AND YOUR
METER LEVEL YOU FELT AFTER EATING. REMEMBER TO HAVE AN
ADEQUATE AMOUNT OF PROTEIN TO SUSTAIN SATIETY (FEELING
FULLER LONGER), CHOOSE THE GOOD FATS, CHOOSE THE GOOD
CARBS AS YOU GO.

Time	Food & Drink Intake	Cal/Carbs/Sugar/Other	Meter Level
			>HUNGRY
			>FULL
			>JUST STUFFED

NIGHT WEIGHT

MORNING WEIGHT

DATE - DAILY FOOD JOURNAL

FULL BELLY METER WORKBOOK

RECORD THE TIME, ITEM, ANY COUNTS YOU ARE DOING, AND YOUR METER LEVEL YOU FELT AFTER EATING. REMEMBER TO HAVE AN ADEQUATE AMOUNT OF PROTEIN TO SUSTAIN SATIETY (FEELING FULLER LONGER), CHOOSE THE GOOD FATS, CHOOSE THE GOOD CARBS AS YOU GO.

Time	Food & Drink Intake	Cal/Carbs/Sugar/Other	Meter Level
			>HUNGRY
			>FULL
			>JUST STUFFED

NIGHT WEIGHT

MORNING WEIGHT

DATE - DAILY FOOD JOURNAL

FULL BELLY METER WORKBOOK

RECORD THE TIME, ITEM, ANY COUNTS YOU ARE DOING, AND YOUR METER LEVEL YOU FELT AFTER EATING. REMEMBER TO HAVE AN ADEQUATE AMOUNT OF PROTEIN TO SUSTAIN SATIETY (FEELING FULLER LONGER), CHOOSE THE GOOD FATS, CHOOSE THE GOOD CARBS AS YOU GO.

Time	Food & Drink Intake	Cal/Carbs/Sugar/Other	Meter Level
			>HUNGRY
			>FULL
			>JUST STUFFED

NIGHT WEIGHT

MORNING WEIGHT

DATE - DAILY FOOD JOURNAL

FULL BELLY METER WORKBOOK

RECORD THE TIME, ITEM, ANY COUNTS YOU ARE DOING, AND YOUR METER LEVEL YOU FELT AFTER EATING. REMEMBER TO HAVE AN ADEQUATE AMOUNT OF PROTEIN TO SUSTAIN SATIETY (FEELING FULLER LONGER), CHOOSE THE GOOD FATS, CHOOSE THE GOOD CARBS AS YOU GO.

Time	Food & Drink Intake	Cal/Carbs/Sugar/Other	Meter Level
			>HUNGRY
			>FULL
			>JUST STUFFED

NIGHT WEIGHT

MORNING WEIGHT

DATE - DAILY FOOD JOURNAL

FULL BELLY METER WORKBOOK

RECORD THE TIME, ITEM, ANY COUNTS YOU ARE DOING, AND YOUR METER LEVEL YOU FELT AFTER EATING. REMEMBER TO HAVE AN ADEQUATE AMOUNT OF PROTEIN TO SUSTAIN SATIETY (FEELING FULLER LONGER), CHOOSE THE GOOD FATS, CHOOSE THE GOOD CARBS AS YOU GO.

Time	Food & Drink Intake	Cal/Carbs/Sugar/Other	Meter Level
			>HUNGRY
			>FULL
			>JUST STUFFED

NIGHT WEIGHT

_____
MORNING WEIGHT

_____
DATE - DAILY FOOD JOURNAL

FULL BELLY METER WORKBOOK

RECORD THE TIME, ITEM, ANY COUNTS YOU ARE DOING, AND YOUR
METER LEVEL YOU FELT AFTER EATING. REMEMBER TO HAVE AN
ADEQUATE AMOUNT OF PROTEIN TO SUSTAIN SATIETY (FEELING
FULLER LONGER), CHOOSE THE GOOD FATS, CHOOSE THE GOOD
CARBS AS YOU GO.

Time	Food & Drink Intake	Cal/Carbs/Sugar/Other	Meter Level
			›HUNGRY
			›FULL
			›JUST STUFFED

_____
NIGHT WEIGHT

_____   _____
MORNING WEIGHT   DATE - DAILY FOOD JOURNAL

FULL BELLY METER WORKBOOK

RECORD THE TIME, ITEM, ANY COUNTS YOU ARE DOING, AND YOUR
METER LEVEL YOU FELT AFTER EATING. REMEMBER TO HAVE AN
ADEQUATE AMOUNT OF PROTEIN TO SUSTAIN SATIETY (FEELING
FULLER LONGER), CHOOSE THE GOOD FATS, CHOOSE THE GOOD
CARBS AS YOU GO.

Time	Food & Drink Intake	Cal/Carbs/Sugar/Other	Meter Level
			>HUNGRY
			>FULL
			>JUST STUFFED

_____
NIGHT WEIGHT

MORNING WEIGHT

DATE - DAILY FOOD JOURNAL

FULL BELLY METER WORKBOOK

RECORD THE TIME, ITEM, ANY COUNTS YOU ARE DOING, AND YOUR METER LEVEL YOU FELT AFTER EATING. REMEMBER TO HAVE AN ADEQUATE AMOUNT OF PROTEIN TO SUSTAIN SATIETY (FEELING FULLER LONGER), CHOOSE THE GOOD FATS, CHOOSE THE GOOD CARBS AS YOU GO.

Time	Food & Drink Intake	Cal/Carbs/Sugar/Other	Meter Level
			>HUNGRY
			>FULL
			>JUST STUFFED

NIGHT WEIGHT

MORNING WEIGHT

DATE - DAILY FOOD JOURNAL

FULL BELLY METER WORKBOOK

RECORD THE TIME, ITEM, ANY COUNTS YOU ARE DOING, AND YOUR
METER LEVEL YOU FELT AFTER EATING. REMEMBER TO HAVE AN
ADEQUATE AMOUNT OF PROTEIN TO SUSTAIN SATIETY (FEELING
FULLER LONGER), CHOOSE THE GOOD FATS, CHOOSE THE GOOD
CARBS AS YOU GO.

Time	Food & Drink Intake	Cal/Carbs/Sugar/Other	Meter Level
			>HUNGRY
			>FULL
			>JUST STUFFED

NIGHT WEIGHT

_____   _____
MORNING WEIGHT   DATE - DAILY FOOD JOURNAL

FULL BELLY METER WORKBOOK

RECORD THE TIME, ITEM, ANY COUNTS YOU ARE DOING, AND YOUR
METER LEVEL YOU FELT AFTER EATING. REMEMBER TO HAVE AN
ADEQUATE AMOUNT OF PROTEIN TO SUSTAIN SATIETY (FEELING
FULLER LONGER), CHOOSE THE GOOD FATS, CHOOSE THE GOOD
CARBS AS YOU GO.

Time	Food & Drink Intake	Cal/Carbs/Sugar/Other	Meter Level
			>HUNGRY
			>FULL
			>JUST STUFFED

_____
NIGHT WEIGHT

MORNING WEIGHT

DATE - DAILY FOOD JOURNAL

FULL BELLY METER WORKBOOK

RECORD THE TIME, ITEM, ANY COUNTS YOU ARE DOING, AND YOUR METER LEVEL YOU FELT AFTER EATING. REMEMBER TO HAVE AN ADEQUATE AMOUNT OF PROTEIN TO SUSTAIN SATIETY (FEELING FULLER LONGER), CHOOSE THE GOOD FATS, CHOOSE THE GOOD CARBS AS YOU GO.

Time	Food & Drink Intake	Cal/Carbs/Sugar/Other	Meter Level
			>HUNGRY
			>FULL
			>JUST STUFFED

NIGHT WEIGHT

MORNING WEIGHT

DATE - DAILY FOOD JOURNAL

FULL BELLY METER WORKBOOK

RECORD THE TIME, ITEM, ANY COUNTS YOU ARE DOING, AND YOUR
METER LEVEL YOU FELT AFTER EATING. REMEMBER TO HAVE AN
ADEQUATE AMOUNT OF PROTEIN TO SUSTAIN SATIETY (FEELING
FULLER LONGER), CHOOSE THE GOOD FATS, CHOOSE THE GOOD
CARBS AS YOU GO.

Time	Food & Drink Intake	Cal/Carbs/Sugar/Other	Meter Level
			>HUNGRY
			>FULL
			>JUST STUFFED

NIGHT WEIGHT

MORNING WEIGHT

DATE - DAILY FOOD JOURNAL

FULL BELLY METER WORKBOOK

RECORD THE TIME, ITEM, ANY COUNTS YOU ARE DOING, AND YOUR METER LEVEL YOU FELT AFTER EATING. REMEMBER TO HAVE AN ADEQUATE AMOUNT OF PROTEIN TO SUSTAIN SATIETY (FEELING FULLER LONGER), CHOOSE THE GOOD FATS, CHOOSE THE GOOD CARBS AS YOU GO.

Time	Food & Drink Intake	Cal/Carbs/Sugar/Other	Meter Level
			>HUNGRY >FULL >JUST STUFFED

NIGHT WEIGHT

_____
MORNING WEIGHT

_____
DATE - DAILY FOOD JOURNAL

FULL BELLY METER WORKBOOK

RECORD THE TIME, ITEM, ANY COUNTS YOU ARE DOING, AND YOUR
METER LEVEL YOU FELT AFTER EATING. REMEMBER TO HAVE AN
ADEQUATE AMOUNT OF PROTEIN TO SUSTAIN SATIETY (FEELING
FULLER LONGER), CHOOSE THE GOOD FATS, CHOOSE THE GOOD
CARBS AS YOU GO.

Time	Food & Drink Intake	Cal/Carbs/Sugar/Other	Meter Level
			>HUNGRY
			>FULL
			>JUST STUFFED

_____
NIGHT WEIGHT

MORNING WEIGHT

DATE - DAILY FOOD JOURNAL

FULL BELLY METER WORKBOOK

RECORD THE TIME, ITEM, ANY COUNTS YOU ARE DOING, AND YOUR METER LEVEL YOU FELT AFTER EATING. REMEMBER TO HAVE AN ADEQUATE AMOUNT OF PROTEIN TO SUSTAIN SATIETY (FEELING FULLER LONGER), CHOOSE THE GOOD FATS, CHOOSE THE GOOD CARBS AS YOU GO.

Time	Food & Drink Intake	Cal/Carbs/Sugar/Other	Meter Level
			>HUNGRY
			>FULL
			>JUST STUFFED

NIGHT WEIGHT

MORNING WEIGHT

DATE - DAILY FOOD JOURNAL

FULL BELLY METER WORKBOOK

RECORD THE TIME, ITEM, ANY COUNTS YOU ARE DOING, AND YOUR METER LEVEL YOU FELT AFTER EATING. REMEMBER TO HAVE AN ADEQUATE AMOUNT OF PROTEIN TO SUSTAIN SATIETY (FEELING FULLER LONGER), CHOOSE THE GOOD FATS, CHOOSE THE GOOD CARBS AS YOU GO.

Time	Food & Drink Intake	Cal/Carbs/Sugar/Other	Meter Level
			>HUNGRY
			>FULL
			>JUST STUFFED

NIGHT WEIGHT

MORNING WEIGHT

DATE - DAILY FOOD JOURNAL

FULL BELLY METER WORKBOOK

RECORD THE TIME, ITEM, ANY COUNTS YOU ARE DOING, AND YOUR METER LEVEL YOU FELT AFTER EATING. REMEMBER TO HAVE AN ADEQUATE AMOUNT OF PROTEIN TO SUSTAIN SATIETY (FEELING FULLER LONGER), CHOOSE THE GOOD FATS, CHOOSE THE GOOD CARBS AS YOU GO.

Time	Food & Drink Intake	Cal/Carbs/Sugar/Other	Meter Level
			>HUNGRY
			>FULL
			>JUST STUFFED

NIGHT WEIGHT

MORNING WEIGHT

DATE - DAILY FOOD JOURNAL

FULL BELLY METER WORKBOOK

RECORD THE TIME, ITEM, ANY COUNTS YOU ARE DOING, AND YOUR
METER LEVEL YOU FELT AFTER EATING. REMEMBER TO HAVE AN
ADEQUATE AMOUNT OF PROTEIN TO SUSTAIN SATIETY (FEELING
FULLER LONGER), CHOOSE THE GOOD FATS, CHOOSE THE GOOD
CARBS AS YOU GO.

Time	Food & Drink Intake	Cal/Carbs/Sugar/Other	Meter Level
			›HUNGRY
			›FULL
			›JUST STUFFED

NIGHT WEIGHT

MORNING WEIGHT

DATE - DAILY FOOD JOURNAL

FULL BELLY METER WORKBOOK

RECORD THE TIME, ITEM, ANY COUNTS YOU ARE DOING, AND YOUR
METER LEVEL YOU FELT AFTER EATING. REMEMBER TO HAVE AN
ADEQUATE AMOUNT OF PROTEIN TO SUSTAIN SATIETY (FEELING
FULLER LONGER), CHOOSE THE GOOD FATS, CHOOSE THE GOOD
CARBS AS YOU GO.

Time	Food & Drink Intake	Cal/Carbs/Sugar/Other	Meter Level
			>HUNGRY
			>FULL
			>JUST STUFFED

NIGHT WEIGHT

MORNING WEIGHT

DATE - DAILY FOOD JOURNAL

FULL BELLY METER WORKBOOK

RECORD THE TIME, ITEM, ANY COUNTS YOU ARE DOING, AND YOUR METER LEVEL YOU FELT AFTER EATING. REMEMBER TO HAVE AN ADEQUATE AMOUNT OF PROTEIN TO SUSTAIN SATIETY (FEELING FULLER LONGER), CHOOSE THE GOOD FATS, CHOOSE THE GOOD CARBS AS YOU GO.

Time	Food & Drink Intake	Cal/Carbs/Sugar/Other	Meter Level
			>HUNGRY
			>FULL
			>JUST STUFFED

NIGHT WEIGHT

MORNING WEIGHT

DATE - DAILY FOOD JOURNAL

FULL BELLY METER WORKBOOK

RECORD THE TIME, ITEM, ANY COUNTS YOU ARE DOING, AND YOUR
METER LEVEL YOU FELT AFTER EATING. REMEMBER TO HAVE AN
ADEQUATE AMOUNT OF PROTEIN TO SUSTAIN SATIETY (FEELING
FULLER LONGER), CHOOSE THE GOOD FATS, CHOOSE THE GOOD
CARBS AS YOU GO.

Time	Food & Drink Intake	Cal/Carbs/Sugar/Other	Meter Level
			>HUNGRY
			>FULL
			>JUST STUFFED

NIGHT WEIGHT

MORNING WEIGHT

DATE - DAILY FOOD JOURNAL

FULL BELLY METER WORKBOOK

RECORD THE TIME, ITEM, ANY COUNTS YOU ARE DOING, AND YOUR
METER LEVEL YOU FELT AFTER EATING. REMEMBER TO HAVE AN
ADEQUATE AMOUNT OF PROTEIN TO SUSTAIN SATIETY (FEELING
FULLER LONGER), CHOOSE THE GOOD FATS, CHOOSE THE GOOD
CARBS AS YOU GO.

Time	Food & Drink Intake	Cal/Carbs/Sugar/Other	Meter Level
			>HUNGRY
			>FULL
			>JUST STUFFED

NIGHT WEIGHT

MORNING WEIGHT

DATE - DAILY FOOD JOURNAL

FULL BELLY METER WORKBOOK

RECORD THE TIME, ITEM, ANY COUNTS YOU ARE DOING, AND YOUR METER LEVEL YOU FELT AFTER EATING. REMEMBER TO HAVE AN ADEQUATE AMOUNT OF PROTEIN TO SUSTAIN SATIETY (FEELING FULLER LONGER), CHOOSE THE GOOD FATS, CHOOSE THE GOOD CARBS AS YOU GO.

Time	Food & Drink Intake	Cal/Carbs/Sugar/Other	Meter Level
			>HUNGRY
			>FULL
			>JUST STUFFED

NIGHT WEIGHT

MORNING WEIGHT

DATE - DAILY FOOD JOURNAL

FULL BELLY METER WORKBOOK

RECORD THE TIME, ITEM, ANY COUNTS YOU ARE DOING, AND YOUR
METER LEVEL YOU FELT AFTER EATING. REMEMBER TO HAVE AN
ADEQUATE AMOUNT OF PROTEIN TO SUSTAIN SATIETY (FEELING
FULLER LONGER), CHOOSE THE GOOD FATS, CHOOSE THE GOOD
CARBS AS YOU GO.

Time	Food & Drink Intake	Cal/Carbs/Sugar/Other	Meter Level
			›HUNGRY
			›FULL
			›JUST STUFFED

NIGHT WEIGHT

MORNING WEIGHT

DATE - DAILY FOOD JOURNAL

FULL BELLY METER WORKBOOK

RECORD THE TIME, ITEM, ANY COUNTS YOU ARE DOING, AND YOUR
METER LEVEL YOU FELT AFTER EATING. REMEMBER TO HAVE AN
ADEQUATE AMOUNT OF PROTEIN TO SUSTAIN SATIETY (FEELING
FULLER LONGER), CHOOSE THE GOOD FATS, CHOOSE THE GOOD
CARBS AS YOU GO.

Time	Food & Drink Intake	Cal/Carbs/Sugar/Other	Meter Level
			>HUNGRY
			>FULL
			>JUST STUFFED

NIGHT WEIGHT

MORNING WEIGHT

DATE - DAILY FOOD JOURNAL

FULL BELLY METER WORKBOOK

RECORD THE TIME, ITEM, ANY COUNTS YOU ARE DOING, AND YOUR METER LEVEL YOU FELT AFTER EATING. REMEMBER TO HAVE AN ADEQUATE AMOUNT OF PROTEIN TO SUSTAIN SATIETY (FEELING FULLER LONGER), CHOOSE THE GOOD FATS, CHOOSE THE GOOD CARBS AS YOU GO.

Time	Food & Drink Intake	Cal/Carbs/Sugar/Other	Meter Level
			>HUNGRY
			>FULL
			>JUST STUFFED

NIGHT WEIGHT

MORNING WEIGHT

DATE - DAILY FOOD JOURNAL

FULL BELLY METER WORKBOOK

RECORD THE TIME, ITEM, ANY COUNTS YOU ARE DOING, AND YOUR METER LEVEL YOU FELT AFTER EATING. REMEMBER TO HAVE AN ADEQUATE AMOUNT OF PROTEIN TO SUSTAIN SATIETY (FEELING FULLER LONGER), CHOOSE THE GOOD FATS, CHOOSE THE GOOD CARBS AS YOU GO.

Time	Food & Drink Intake	Cal/Carbs/Sugar/Other	Meter Level
			>HUNGRY
			>FULL
			>JUST STUFFED

NIGHT WEIGHT

MORNING WEIGHT

DATE - DAILY FOOD JOURNAL

FULL BELLY METER WORKBOOK

RECORD THE TIME, ITEM, ANY COUNTS YOU ARE DOING, AND YOUR METER LEVEL YOU FELT AFTER EATING. REMEMBER TO HAVE AN ADEQUATE AMOUNT OF PROTEIN TO SUSTAIN SATIETY (FEELING FULLER LONGER), CHOOSE THE GOOD FATS, CHOOSE THE GOOD CARBS AS YOU GO.

Time	Food & Drink Intake	Cal/Carbs/Sugar/Other	Meter Level
			>HUNGRY
			>FULL
			>JUST STUFFED

NIGHT WEIGHT

MORNING WEIGHT

DATE - DAILY FOOD JOURNAL

FULL BELLY METER WORKBOOK

RECORD THE TIME, ITEM, ANY COUNTS YOU ARE DOING, AND YOUR METER LEVEL YOU FELT AFTER EATING. REMEMBER TO HAVE AN ADEQUATE AMOUNT OF PROTEIN TO SUSTAIN SATIETY (FEELING FULLER LONGER), CHOOSE THE GOOD FATS, CHOOSE THE GOOD CARBS AS YOU GO.

Time	Food & Drink Intake	Cal/Carbs/Sugar/Other	Meter Level
			>HUNGRY
			>FULL
			>JUST STUFFED

NIGHT WEIGHT

MORNING WEIGHT

DATE - DAILY FOOD JOURNAL

FULL BELLY METER WORKBOOK

RECORD THE TIME, ITEM, ANY COUNTS YOU ARE DOING, AND YOUR METER LEVEL YOU FELT AFTER EATING. REMEMBER TO HAVE AN ADEQUATE AMOUNT OF PROTEIN TO SUSTAIN SATIETY (FEELING FULLER LONGER), CHOOSE THE GOOD FATS, CHOOSE THE GOOD CARBS AS YOU GO.

Time	Food & Drink Intake	Cal/Carbs/Sugar/Other	Meter Level
			›HUNGRY
			›FULL
			›JUST STUFFED

NIGHT WEIGHT

MORNING WEIGHT

DATE - DAILY FOOD JOURNAL

FULL BELLY METER WORKBOOK

RECORD THE TIME, ITEM, ANY COUNTS YOU ARE DOING, AND YOUR
METER LEVEL YOU FELT AFTER EATING. REMEMBER TO HAVE AN
ADEQUATE AMOUNT OF PROTEIN TO SUSTAIN SATIETY (FEELING
FULLER LONGER), CHOOSE THE GOOD FATS, CHOOSE THE GOOD
CARBS AS YOU GO.

Time	Food & Drink Intake	Cal/Carbs/Sugar/Other	Meter Level
			>HUNGRY
			>FULL
			>JUST STUFFED

NIGHT WEIGHT

MORNING WEIGHT

DATE - DAILY FOOD JOURNAL

FULL BELLY METER WORKBOOK

RECORD THE TIME, ITEM, ANY COUNTS YOU ARE DOING, AND YOUR METER LEVEL YOU FELT AFTER EATING. REMEMBER TO HAVE AN ADEQUATE AMOUNT OF PROTEIN TO SUSTAIN SATIETY (FEELING FULLER LONGER), CHOOSE THE GOOD FATS, CHOOSE THE GOOD CARBS AS YOU GO.

Time	Food & Drink Intake	Cal/Carbs/Sugar/Other	Meter Level
			>HUNGRY
			>FULL
			>JUST STUFFED

NIGHT WEIGHT

MORNING WEIGHT

DATE - DAILY FOOD JOURNAL

FULL BELLY METER WORKBOOK

RECORD THE TIME, ITEM, ANY COUNTS YOU ARE DOING, AND YOUR
METER LEVEL YOU FELT AFTER EATING. REMEMBER TO HAVE AN
ADEQUATE AMOUNT OF PROTEIN TO SUSTAIN SATIETY (FEELING
FULLER LONGER), CHOOSE THE GOOD FATS, CHOOSE THE GOOD
CARBS AS YOU GO.

Time	Food & Drink Intake	Cal/Carbs/Sugar/Other	Meter Level
			>HUNGRY
			>FULL
			>JUST STUFFED

NIGHT WEIGHT

MORNING WEIGHT

DATE - DAILY FOOD JOURNAL

FULL BELLY METER WORKBOOK

RECORD THE TIME, ITEM, ANY COUNTS YOU ARE DOING, AND YOUR
METER LEVEL YOU FELT AFTER EATING. REMEMBER TO HAVE AN
ADEQUATE AMOUNT OF PROTEIN TO SUSTAIN SATIETY (FEELING
FULLER LONGER), CHOOSE THE GOOD FATS, CHOOSE THE GOOD
CARBS AS YOU GO.

Time	Food & Drink Intake	Cal/Carbs/Sugar/Other	Meter Level
			›HUNGRY
			›FULL
			›JUST STUFFED

NIGHT WEIGHT

_____
MORNING WEIGHT

_____
DATE - DAILY FOOD JOURNAL

FULL BELLY METER WORKBOOK

RECORD THE TIME, ITEM, ANY COUNTS YOU ARE DOING, AND YOUR
METER LEVEL YOU FELT AFTER EATING. REMEMBER TO HAVE AN
ADEQUATE AMOUNT OF PROTEIN TO SUSTAIN SATIETY (FEELING
FULLER LONGER), CHOOSE THE GOOD FATS, CHOOSE THE GOOD
CARBS AS YOU GO.

Time	Food & Drink Intake	Cal/Carbs/Sugar/Other	Meter Level
			>HUNGRY
			>FULL
			>JUST STUFFED

_____
NIGHT WEIGHT

_____   _____
MORNING WEIGHT   DATE - DAILY FOOD JOURNAL

FULL BELLY METER WORKBOOK

RECORD THE TIME, ITEM, ANY COUNTS YOU ARE DOING, AND YOUR
METER LEVEL YOU FELT AFTER EATING. REMEMBER TO HAVE AN
ADEQUATE AMOUNT OF PROTEIN TO SUSTAIN SATIETY (FEELING
FULLER LONGER), CHOOSE THE GOOD FATS, CHOOSE THE GOOD
CARBS AS YOU GO.

Time	Food & Drink Intake	Cal/Carbs/Sugar/Other	Meter Level
			>HUNGRY
			>FULL
			>JUST STUFFED

_____
NIGHT WEIGHT

MORNING WEIGHT

DATE - DAILY FOOD JOURNAL

FULL BELLY METER WORKBOOK

RECORD THE TIME, ITEM, ANY COUNTS YOU ARE DOING, AND YOUR
METER LEVEL YOU FELT AFTER EATING. REMEMBER TO HAVE AN
ADEQUATE AMOUNT OF PROTEIN TO SUSTAIN SATIETY (FEELING
FULLER LONGER), CHOOSE THE GOOD FATS, CHOOSE THE GOOD
CARBS AS YOU GO.

Time	Food & Drink Intake	Cal/Carbs/Sugar/Other	Meter Level
			>HUNGRY >FULL >JUST STUFFED

NIGHT WEIGHT

MORNING WEIGHT

DATE - DAILY FOOD JOURNAL

FULL BELLY METER WORKBOOK

RECORD THE TIME, ITEM, ANY COUNTS YOU ARE DOING, AND YOUR
METER LEVEL YOU FELT AFTER EATING. REMEMBER TO HAVE AN
ADEQUATE AMOUNT OF PROTEIN TO SUSTAIN SATIETY (FEELING
FULLER LONGER), CHOOSE THE GOOD FATS, CHOOSE THE GOOD
CARBS AS YOU GO.

Time	Food & Drink Intake	Cal/Carbs/Sugar/Other	Meter Level
			>HUNGRY
			>FULL
			>JUST STUFFED

NIGHT WEIGHT

_____
MORNING WEIGHT

_____
DATE - DAILY FOOD JOURNAL

FULL BELLY METER WORKBOOK

RECORD THE TIME, ITEM, ANY COUNTS YOU ARE DOING, AND YOUR METER LEVEL YOU FELT AFTER EATING. REMEMBER TO HAVE AN ADEQUATE AMOUNT OF PROTEIN TO SUSTAIN SATIETY (FEELING FULLER LONGER), CHOOSE THE GOOD FATS, CHOOSE THE GOOD CARBS AS YOU GO.

Time	Food & Drink Intake	Cal/Carbs/Sugar/Other	Meter Level
			>HUNGRY
			>FULL
			>JUST STUFFED

_____
NIGHT WEIGHT

_____
MORNING WEIGHT

_____
DATE - DAILY FOOD JOURNAL

FULL BELLY METER WORKBOOK

RECORD THE TIME, ITEM, ANY COUNTS YOU ARE DOING, AND YOUR
METER LEVEL YOU FELT AFTER EATING. REMEMBER TO HAVE AN
ADEQUATE AMOUNT OF PROTEIN TO SUSTAIN SATIETY (FEELING
FULLER LONGER), CHOOSE THE GOOD FATS, CHOOSE THE GOOD
CARBS AS YOU GO.

Time	Food & Drink Intake	Cal/Carbs/Sugar/Other	Meter Level
			>HUNGRY
			>FULL
			>JUST STUFFED

_____
NIGHT WEIGHT

MORNING WEIGHT

DATE - DAILY FOOD JOURNAL

FULL BELLY METER WORKBOOK

RECORD THE TIME, ITEM, ANY COUNTS YOU ARE DOING, AND YOUR
METER LEVEL YOU FELT AFTER EATING. REMEMBER TO HAVE AN
ADEQUATE AMOUNT OF PROTEIN TO SUSTAIN SATIETY (FEELING
FULLER LONGER), CHOOSE THE GOOD FATS, CHOOSE THE GOOD
CARBS AS YOU GO.

Time	Food & Drink Intake	Cal/Carbs/Sugar/Other	Meter Level
			>HUNGRY
			>FULL
			>JUST STUFFED

NIGHT WEIGHT

MORNING WEIGHT

DATE - DAILY FOOD JOURNAL

FULL BELLY METER WORKBOOK

RECORD THE TIME, ITEM, ANY COUNTS YOU ARE DOING, AND YOUR METER LEVEL YOU FELT AFTER EATING. REMEMBER TO HAVE AN ADEQUATE AMOUNT OF PROTEIN TO SUSTAIN SATIETY (FEELING FULLER LONGER), CHOOSE THE GOOD FATS, CHOOSE THE GOOD CARBS AS YOU GO.

Time	Food & Drink Intake	Cal/Carbs/Sugar/Other	Meter Level
			›HUNGRY
			›FULL
			›JUST STUFFED

NIGHT WEIGHT

MORNING WEIGHT

DATE - DAILY FOOD JOURNAL

FULL BELLY METER WORKBOOK

RECORD THE TIME, ITEM, ANY COUNTS YOU ARE DOING, AND YOUR
METER LEVEL YOU FELT AFTER EATING. REMEMBER TO HAVE AN
ADEQUATE AMOUNT OF PROTEIN TO SUSTAIN SATIETY (FEELING
FULLER LONGER), CHOOSE THE GOOD FATS, CHOOSE THE GOOD
CARBS AS YOU GO.

Time	Food & Drink Intake	Cal/Carbs/Sugar/Other	Meter Level
			>HUNGRY
			>FULL
			>JUST STUFFED

NIGHT WEIGHT

_____   _____
MORNING WEIGHT   DATE - DAILY FOOD JOURNAL

FULL BELLY METER WORKBOOK

RECORD THE TIME, ITEM, ANY COUNTS YOU ARE DOING, AND YOUR
METER LEVEL YOU FELT AFTER EATING. REMEMBER TO HAVE AN
ADEQUATE AMOUNT OF PROTEIN TO SUSTAIN SATIETY (FEELING
FULLER LONGER), CHOOSE THE GOOD FATS, CHOOSE THE GOOD
CARBS AS YOU GO.

Time	Food & Drink Intake	Cal/Carbs/Sugar/Other	Meter Level
			>HUNGRY
			>FULL
			>JUST STUFFED

_____
NIGHT WEIGHT

MORNING WEIGHT   DATE - DAILY FOOD JOURNAL

FULL BELLY METER WORKBOOK

RECORD THE TIME, ITEM, ANY COUNTS YOU ARE DOING, AND YOUR
METER LEVEL YOU FELT AFTER EATING. REMEMBER TO HAVE AN
ADEQUATE AMOUNT OF PROTEIN TO SUSTAIN SATIETY (FEELING
FULLER LONGER), CHOOSE THE GOOD FATS, CHOOSE THE GOOD
CARBS AS YOU GO.

Time	Food & Drink Intake	Cal/Carbs/Sugar/Other	Meter Level
			>HUNGRY
			>FULL
			>JUST STUFFED

NIGHT WEIGHT

MORNING WEIGHT

DATE - DAILY FOOD JOURNAL

FULL BELLY METER WORKBOOK

RECORD THE TIME, ITEM, ANY COUNTS YOU ARE DOING, AND YOUR METER LEVEL YOU FELT AFTER EATING. REMEMBER TO HAVE AN ADEQUATE AMOUNT OF PROTEIN TO SUSTAIN SATIETY (FEELING FULLER LONGER), CHOOSE THE GOOD FATS, CHOOSE THE GOOD CARBS AS YOU GO.

Time	Food & Drink Intake	Cal/Carbs/Sugar/Other	Meter Level
			›HUNGRY
			›FULL
			›JUST STUFFED

NIGHT WEIGHT

MORNING WEIGHT

DATE - DAILY FOOD JOURNAL

FULL BELLY METER WORKBOOK

RECORD THE TIME, ITEM, ANY COUNTS YOU ARE DOING, AND YOUR
METER LEVEL YOU FELT AFTER EATING. REMEMBER TO HAVE AN
ADEQUATE AMOUNT OF PROTEIN TO SUSTAIN SATIETY (FEELING
FULLER LONGER), CHOOSE THE GOOD FATS, CHOOSE THE GOOD
CARBS AS YOU GO.

Time	Food & Drink Intake	Cal/Carbs/Sugar/Other	Meter Level
			>HUNGRY
			>FULL
			>JUST STUFFED

NIGHT WEIGHT

_____
MORNING WEIGHT

_____
DATE - DAILY FOOD JOURNAL

FULL BELLY METER WORKBOOK

RECORD THE TIME, ITEM, ANY COUNTS YOU ARE DOING, AND YOUR
METER LEVEL YOU FELT AFTER EATING. REMEMBER TO HAVE AN
ADEQUATE AMOUNT OF PROTEIN TO SUSTAIN SATIETY (FEELING
FULLER LONGER), CHOOSE THE GOOD FATS, CHOOSE THE GOOD
CARBS AS YOU GO.

Time	Food & Drink Intake	Cal/Carbs/Sugar/Other	Meter Level
			›HUNGRY
			›FULL
			›JUST STUFFED

_____
NIGHT WEIGHT

MORNING WEIGHT

DATE - DAILY FOOD JOURNAL

FULL BELLY METER WORKBOOK

RECORD THE TIME, ITEM, ANY COUNTS YOU ARE DOING, AND YOUR
METER LEVEL YOU FELT AFTER EATING. REMEMBER TO HAVE AN
ADEQUATE AMOUNT OF PROTEIN TO SUSTAIN SATIETY (FEELING
FULLER LONGER). CHOOSE THE GOOD FATS. CHOOSE THE GOOD
CARBS AS YOU GO.

Time	Food & Drink Intake	Cal/Carbs/Sugar/Other	Meter Level
			›HUNGRY
			›FULL
			›JUST STUFFED

NIGHT WEIGHT

MORNING WEIGHT

DATE - DAILY FOOD JOURNAL

FULL BELLY METER WORKBOOK

RECORD THE TIME, ITEM, ANY COUNTS YOU ARE DOING, AND YOUR METER LEVEL YOU FELT AFTER EATING. REMEMBER TO HAVE AN ADEQUATE AMOUNT OF PROTEIN TO SUSTAIN SATIETY (FEELING FULLER LONGER), CHOOSE THE GOOD FATS, CHOOSE THE GOOD CARBS AS YOU GO.

Time	Food & Drink Intake	Cal/Carbs/Sugar/Other	Meter Level
			>HUNGRY
			>FULL
			>JUST STUFFED

NIGHT WEIGHT

MORNING WEIGHT

DATE - DAILY FOOD JOURNAL

FULL BELLY METER WORKBOOK

RECORD THE TIME, ITEM, ANY COUNTS YOU ARE DOING, AND YOUR METER LEVEL YOU FELT AFTER EATING. REMEMBER TO HAVE AN ADEQUATE AMOUNT OF PROTEIN TO SUSTAIN SATIETY (FEELING FULLER LONGER), CHOOSE THE GOOD FATS, CHOOSE THE GOOD CARBS AS YOU GO.

Time	Food & Drink Intake	Cal/Carbs/Sugar/Other	Meter Level
			>HUNGRY
			>FULL
			>JUST STUFFED

NIGHT WEIGHT

MORNING WEIGHT

DATE - DAILY FOOD JOURNAL

FULL BELLY METER WORKBOOK

RECORD THE TIME, ITEM, ANY COUNTS YOU ARE DOING, AND YOUR
METER LEVEL YOU FELT AFTER EATING. REMEMBER TO HAVE AN
ADEQUATE AMOUNT OF PROTEIN TO SUSTAIN SATIETY (FEELING
FULLER LONGER), CHOOSE THE GOOD FATS, CHOOSE THE GOOD
CARBS AS YOU GO.

Time	Food & Drink Intake	Cal/Carbs/Sugar/Other	Meter Level
			>HUNGRY
			>FULL
			>JUST STUFFED

NIGHT WEIGHT

MORNING WEIGHT

DATE - DAILY FOOD JOURNAL

FULL BELLY METER WORKBOOK

RECORD THE TIME, ITEM, ANY COUNTS YOU ARE DOING, AND YOUR METER LEVEL YOU FELT AFTER EATING. REMEMBER TO HAVE AN ADEQUATE AMOUNT OF PROTEIN TO SUSTAIN SATIETY (FEELING FULLER LONGER), CHOOSE THE GOOD FATS, CHOOSE THE GOOD CARBS AS YOU GO.

Time	Food & Drink Intake	Cal/Carbs/Sugar/Other	Meter Level
			>HUNGRY
			>FULL
			>JUST STUFFED

NIGHT WEIGHT

MY NOTES

MY NOTES

www.ingramcontent.com/pod-product-compliance
Lightning Source LLC
Chambersburg PA
CBHW070911270326
41927CB00011B/2531